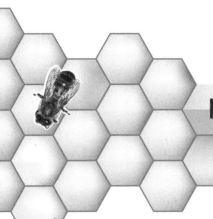

Foundations in Nursing and Health Care

Writing Skills in Health Care

Philip Burnard
Series Editor: Lynne Wigens

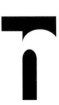

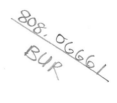

A version of this book was previously published under the title of *Writing for health
professionals: a manual for writers*.

Published in 2004 by:
Nelson Thornes Ltd
Delta Place
27 Bath Road
CHELTENHAM
GL53 7TH
United Kingdom

03 04 05 06 07 / 10 9 8 7 6 5 4 3 2 1

A catalogue record for this book is available from the British Library

ISBN 0 7487 7545 5

Illustrations by Clinton Banbury
Page make-up by Florence Production Ltd

Printed in Great Britain by Ashford Colour Press

Contents

Acknowledgements

Many people have been helpful in the preparation of this book. Thanks go to Helen Broadfield, Sukie Hunter and Helen Kerindi at Nelson Thornes. Particular thanks go to Gareth Marshall for his help with the chapters on computing and software. As always, thanks to my family, Sally, Aaron and Rebecca for their support and patience.

Preface

I try to leave out the parts that people skip.

Elmore Leonard

Like it or not, students, nurses and health professionals have to write. In the last few years, this has become even more apparent. As health professionals of all sorts become more highly qualified, so students have to write more. Many write essays and projects for courses, others carry out research projects and many more share their ideas through writing for publication. With the continuing development of the Internet – that sprawling but useful network of computer networks – many people are writing in a new, immediate way. The Internet allows health professionals to communicate around the world in seconds. It seems unlikely, though, that the Internet will completely replace the more formal written word: in papers, articles, books and records.

Non-fiction writing is more attractive when it is easy to read. It helps everyone if what you write is both easy and interesting to look at. Most of us can improve our writing. I have tried to make this a practical book about writing. For the sort of writing that health professionals most often do is of a *practical* nature. This book, then, is about non-fiction writing – writing so that students, health professionals, teachers, patients and anyone else with whom we come in contact can make sense of what we think and do.

When you write a book like this you put yourself on the line. You run the risk of people reading what you have written and saying 'He is saying one thing and doing another'. You stand to break the rules that you set up – quite badly. That is probably not such a terrible thing. Besides, that should be part of the process of using this book. As you read it, notice when rules are broken. Check the phrasing, the sentence and paragraph construction and see whether or not I have stuck to the rules. Then see whether or not the rules would have improved the passage in question. Begin to read books as much for their style, layout and general format as for their content. If you are going to write, you need to see plenty of examples of all of these things: good, bad and indifferent.

A word about sexism and the writing process. I find the use of 'his or her' and its variants clumsy. I have decided to use 'her' to refer to the person who might be writing, throughout the book. Read 'his' where this applies to you. At present, there is no elegant way of avoiding sexism in writing but we should continue to work at it.

Who is the book for?

All students and health professionals have to write. Some enjoy doing it. Others loathe the thought of picking up a pen or sitting at a keyboard. This book is for a wide range of health professionals. In particular, I hope it will be of use to the following groups of people:

- Students in the health professions on certificate, diploma, undergraduate and postgraduate courses
- Student researchers who have to write papers, dissertations or theses
- Practitioners in the clinical or community field who find themselves wanting or having to write
- Managers who have to prepare reports and are not sure how to
- Lecturers and teachers who want some ideas about advising students
- The general reader who wants some straightforward ideas about how to write.

In a phrase: this book is for you. If you want to write, it will give you some practical help. It won't make writing easy, if you already find it difficult. But it might help.

What is in the book?

In summary, this book aims to help you do the following things:

- Write clearly and well
- Keep a bibliographic database
- Write essays
- Write articles
- Write books
- Write reviews
- Write research reports, dissertations and theses

- Choose a computer for writing
- Select the right software
- Use computers as an aid to writing
- Lay out and edit your work.

While almost anyone can write, there are certain rules that can make writing easier. Also, there are two keywords that I will often return to in this book. They are: *structure* and *simplicity*. If you want to write well, structure your work. If you want to be understood and want people to enjoy reading your work, keep it simple. Look at literature. Most modern literature is simply written. The most difficult things can be understood more easily if they are written clearly and simply.* Think about it. If it can be said at all, it can be said clearly. If it cannot be said, we are better off not trying to say it. That seems to me to sum up the issue.

Here, already, is an indication of the sort of observation I would like you to make. In the last paragraph, I used a footnote. Footnotes are not very popular these days and for good reason. Notice what the footnote made you do. You had to look down to the bottom of the page. In doing so, you probably lost your place and had to find it again. You probably forgot what I was writing about. First lesson: avoid footnotes like the plague. Also, avoid tired clichés. Unfortunately, you will note that I break both of these rules. That may be the second lesson: break the rules occasionally.

The first chapter deals with the basics: how to begin to write and how to structure your work. Then there is a chapter on the basic equipment you might need. The next two deal with the question of computing. Chapter 5 tells you how to set up and use computer databases as an aid to writing. The following chapters consider specific sorts of writing: essays, theses and dissertations, articles and books. You may find, once you start writing, that you progress through these different levels. You may, for example, start by having to write essays for a course. You might then write a very good one that someone advises you to send in for publication. Then, rather than taking the person at her word, you have work to do. You cannot just send in the essay as it stands. Chapter 9 will tell you how to modify it so that it might be published. There is a big difference between writing essays and writing articles. In Chapter 11, I explain how I write and hope that this summarises what has gone before.

---

*Wittgenstein, the philosopher, put this into one of his major philosophical works: that which can be stated can be stated clearly: that of which we cannot speak we should pass over in silence (Wittgenstein 1961).

If you get articles published, you may want to try writing a book. The health-care field is a large one and there is always room for a new approach to an aspect of it. A book turns out to be like an article, only bigger. How much bigger? Read Chapter 10 and you will find out. Again, you will also find how structure can help to make your ideas into a book.

I hope that this book will help you in whatever sort of writing you have to do.

How do I use the book?

There are at least two ways to read this book. One is to start at the beginning and work your way through. This is obviously true of any book. So obviously true that many people think that this is the proper way to read a book. It is if the book is a novel. With non-fiction, though, it is often more useful to browse through the contents page and the index and then to decide which parts of the book you are going to find most useful. Most non-fiction is best read in this way. It is rarely helpful to sit down (or worse – lie down) and read such a book from cover to cover. Instead, read selectively. I usually find that when I begin to read a book in this way I end up reading the whole book: but not in the order that the writer put the chapters together.

Also, if this is your book, make liberal use of a marker pen. Highlight the passages that are going to help you when you get down to your own writing. In the end, books are for using. That is why paperbacks are so much better than hardbacks. People are less reverent towards them. This can have at least two effects. First, readers are less likely to think that 'it must be right because it's in a book' – people become more critical.

Second, readers are less likely to feel that they must not write in the paragraphs or use marker pens. The reason that you can buy so many different sorts of marker pen is simply because there is a market for them. Buy a whole range and use them liberally. Only do this if you own the book. I hate bringing home library books and finding that a previous reader has added her own comments. Sometimes they are humorous in their extremity (awful book! don't read this page!) but in the end, they are annoying. Do write in your own books.

I have enjoyed writing and rewriting this book and I have learned a lot about writing in the process. I hope that you find it useful and wish you the best of luck with your own writing projects. Start writing now.

Philip Burnard

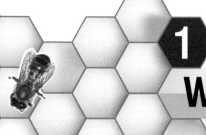

1

Writing: the basics

Learning outcomes

By the end of this chapter you should be able to:

- Understand the effects of layout and punctuation in your writing
- Know how to keep your writing clear and simple
- Begin developing your own writing routine: when, where, how.

My task is by the power of the written word to make you hear, to make you feel – it is, before all, to make you see.

Joseph Conrad

I notice that you use plain, simple language, short words and brief sentences. That is the way to write English. It is the modern way and the best way. Stick to it.

Mark Twain

An author called Ernest Gaines once wrote what he called the 'Six Golden Rules of Writing': read, read, read and write, write, write. These simple rules are hard to better. The writer must read. Reading is the fuel for good writing whatever the writing might be for. If you are a health professional who is intending to write, it is likely that you already read. But what do you read? Novels? Textbooks? Research reports? Papers that you are referred to by your colleagues or teachers? The writer reads anything and everything. I think a good starting point for reading is to consider these areas:

- Books related to your field
- Journal papers related to your area of interest
- Peripheral papers
- Magazines related to your field
- Newspapers
- Novels – especially literature
- Autobiographies
- Biographies
- Cereal packets and adverts.

In other words, try to read everything. It is all important fuel however well or badly it may be written – and some of the worst writing comes in the academic journals. Be eclectic. Avoid limiting yourself to heavy books and papers in your field. Not only will you get bored but you will also find your own style quickly becomes stilted and dull. Buy the occasional magazine or journal from a field different from your own. When, for example, did you last pick up or buy *The Grocer*? Have you ever read *Cosmopolitan* or *Computer Shopper*? All magazines can teach you something about writing.

Theory Into Practice

All students and all health care professionals need to keep up to date. The best way of doing this is by regularly reading a range of journals. Journals usually contain much more up-to-date information than books.

This does not mean, of course, that you have to be obsessional about the written word. Alan Bennett makes a nice, dry point about those who find themselves too attached to books:

> As for me, while I'm not baffled by books, I can't see how anyone can love them ('He loved books'). I can't see how anyone can 'love literature'. What does that mean?
>
> Bennett 1994

You may not 'love' them, then, but it is important to read them.

This is the first rule: read as much as you can. Read for content. Read for structure and layout. Have a look through this book. Notice how it is laid out. How many blank lines are there between subheadings and text? Have you noticed details like that before? You will in future – if you intend to write. For the aim is to become a technically proficient writer as well as a 'good' writer. That means mastering some simple rules of layout and design and that is what this book will help you with. You may feel that this is obsessional attention to detail. I don't. I once sent in a manuscript to a heavyweight journal. I had made certain corrections to the typed manuscript and I had simply written them in with a pen. A few weeks later I received this dry comment in a letter of acceptance: 'Please pay more attention to the presentation of your manuscripts otherwise you may not be published in this journal again.'

At first, I took offence and got very high handed about the whole thing. What a nerve. Why should I have to be threatened in this way? After a while, though, and after working as a journal reviewer myself, I came to appreciate what that rather direct editor had in mind. Presentation does matter. It is one thing to write ageless prose (and we are not likely to achieve that in a hurry). It is another to make sure that it is offered to the reader in a recognisable form. The more you write, the more important this becomes. Few book publishers will look favourably on a scrappily typed manuscript. It pays to think about what your finished work will look like on the page.

Notice how layout affects you. If you browse through a bookshop, you don't simply look at authors, titles or covers. You open the book and look through the pages. Why do you do that? Not only to pick up the gist of the book but also to see whether or not you like the layout. As you do this you will notice a number of things without really thinking about it. You will feel the quality of the paper. You will notice how large or small the typeface is. You will notice whether or not words are crammed on to the page or laid out with plenty of 'white space'. It is an interesting and obscure fact that good layout in book printing calls for a ratio of 50% text to 50% of white space. This sounds unlikely but turns out to be true of most printed pages. If the page is more crammed with print than this, you are unlikely to find the book attractive.

In my view, American publishers are better at dealing with the question of page layout than are UK publishers. Most American textbooks are studies in how to make the page and chapter look attractive. On the other hand, the British press is catching up fast. These sorts of concerns should become yours.

If you are writing essays for a course, you may feel that this does not apply to you. It does. As a university professor, I have to mark hundreds of essays and papers for publication every year. I always start with the best-looking ones. Not very academic, you may say. Bear in mind that marking usually takes place late in the evening. It pays to humour the person who is marking your work and offer her something she will enjoy reading. It pays to write well and it pays to present your work well.

Key points **Top tips**

Think carefully about the following issues:

- The paper that you print on
- How you lay out your page
- The typeface or 'font' that you use
- The spacing between lines
- How to make your work look uncluttered and clear
- How many paragraphs you have on a page.

Types of writing

There is a wide range of opportunities to write in the health professions. Opportunity is the right word here although some, as we have noted, see writing as a chore. Perhaps, like other skills, we enjoy writing more when we get better at it. Here are some examples of the opportunities to write:

- Essays
- Reflective diaries
- Dissertations
- Theses
- Research reports
- Abstracts
- Journal articles
- Journal papers
- Books
- Letters to the editor of journals
- Short 'fillers' for magazines
- Short articles for newsletters
- Course materials
- Curriculum packages
- Advertising copy.

The principles that are discussed throughout this book are applicable to all of these sorts of writing. If you hate writing, read on. You may get to like it. You may not, of course, but you may get better at it.

Getting ideas

One thing is important here: you must have something to write about. I once borrowed an idea from the American poet Robert Lowell. I walked into a workshop on writing skills and gave the students instructions. All I said was: 'Write something.' Some got on with this straight away. Others struggled to put two or three sentences together. The point is that you can write about anything. In the health professions there is always something to write about. If you cannot get inspired from the business of caring for other people, draw upon one or more of the following sources of inspiration:

- Personal experience
- Working life
- Family and friends

- Unusual experiences
- Holidays
- Reading
- TV
- Radio
- Visits abroad
- Sexual experiences
- Altered states of consciousness (through meditation, etc.)
- Other people's anecdotes
- Conferences
- Accidents
- Odd experiences
- Your imagination
- The future
- The past
- The immediate present
- How you wish things were
- How you wish things were not
- Your beliefs
- Your values
- Your religious beliefs or lack of them.

It should be easy to add to this list. Writing consists mainly of having something to write about, then exercising some basic skills to get the ideas down on paper. I don't believe that there is anything magical about the process, although I appreciate that some people write better and more easily than others.

Quality and meaning

Is some writing *better* than others? In my list of recommended reading I have suggested that, alongside literature and journals, you read cereal packets. I have been asked by some readers if I mean this, for – surely – there are some forms of text that are better than others. From a post-modern point of view, however, there is nothing *but* the text (Docherty 1993). Text is text is text. It is all black marks on white pages. We, as readers, 'invent' the meaning of the text and – if you like – the 'reader writes the text'. This particularly liberal point of view acknowledges that what is common to all forms of writing is words and words arranged on the page. In this sense, then, all writing is an attempt to communicate and there is never only one meaning attached to what is written. As we read Shakespeare, we bring our own meanings to bear. As we read slogans in advertisements, we also 'read in' our own interpretations of what the advertisers meant. All of this makes it difficult to begin to talk about an absolute yardstick for quality in writing.

On the other hand, if we are to discuss 'rules of writing' – and this book is about those – then it is being acknowledged that certain rules are possible. As always, it is useful to take in a range of points of view – about writing as about other things – and the post-modern view can be useful in thinking differently about writing, quality and meaning.

Rules of good writing

Robert Gunning (1968) offers 10 principles of clear writing:

- Keep sentences short
- Prefer the simple to the complex
- Prefer the familiar word
- Avoid unnecessary words
- Put action in your verbs
- Write like you talk
- Use terms your reader can picture
- Tie in with your reader's experience
- Make full use of variety
- Write to express not impress.

It is worth considering each of these in turn. Gunning's work is a readable and important analysis of how to write well.

Keep sentences short

This speaks for itself. Short sentences (and short paragraphs) are easy on the eye and easy to read. Many people lose the thread of long sentences. Try to get into the habit of halving all your sentences that are more than about six or seven words in length. Most people's writing can benefit from editing in this way. Also, avoid too many lists that end in 'and'. Instead, deal with each item separately. On the other hand, don't try to make all your sentences the same length. Too many short sentences can be a distraction. Use two or three short ones and then use a slightly longer one. Vary your sentence and paragraph length a little. If in doubt, though, keep them short.

> ## Over to you
>
> Consider these three examples and see if what I have written makes sense to you:
>
> ### Example 1
> Most people have to write. Many write for courses. I have completed a number of courses. All required essays. Some wanted long essays. Others wanted short. I found the early ones difficult. Writing got easier later on. Now I enjoy writing. Not everyone does. I wonder if you do.
>
> ### Example 2
> It is probably true that most people have to write at some time in their life. Many people have to write essays for courses and they have all sorts of things to consider when they do this: they have to think about planning their work; they have to find somewhere to write and they have to consider how to integrate their work with their social life. While social life is important to most people it should not interfere with your studies and, if you can, you should avoid mixing the pub with your essay writing activities.
>
> ### Example 3
> Most people have to write. Students usually have to write essays for courses. Essay writing, while not difficult, takes some planning. The key issue is outlining. A simple outline can save time. Most people, once they have learned to outline, find that they can write much more easily. Experimentation may be the answer. Try writing with outlines. Try writing without. If you find that the outlining process helps, keep at it. If not, stop.

Example 1 shows the use of short sentences. While it is readable, the style is rather staccato. The second illustrates how long sentences can be awkward and difficult to follow. The third shows the use of both short and longer sentences. Hopefully, the third example is the easiest to read. Also, the sudden use of a very short sentence can be used to heighten dramatic effect. Note, for example, the terse use of the final sentence in example 3.

Look through some of your own work and edit it. Cut out the lists of items separated by commas and shorten some of the sentences. Then read through your work and see whether or not you agree that shorter sentences make for clearer reading.

Prefer the simple to the complex

Do not try to be clever. You readers will not appreciate it. Stick to ordinary words and do not try to confuse. As one lecturer at university told me, 'anyone who has anything interesting to say will not risk being misunderstood'. Some students on courses are tempted to use flowery language in the belief that it will sound 'academic'. Some academics are tempted this way too. This is fine if you are writing an academic monograph to be read by a handful of other people. Most of us are not (and even in a monograph, simple and clear language is to be preferred).

Consider the following two examples of text written about the same subject but in rather different ways.

Example 1
There is a sense in which all of us can appreciate the universality of the human condition. While, in a sense, we are all unique, so too do we share – in very real ways – a variety of features of considerable similitude. In our being grounded in the very substance of humanity we are able to project outwards and reach out to those with whom we share that humanity.

Example 2
We are similar to each other in some ways. In other ways, we are unique. What is personal is also universal.

I suggest that the second example says much the same as the first but is much simpler and easier to understand. The first example is also full of 'academic' redundancies such as 'there is a sense in which' – a phrase that really means very little.

Strong (1991) says this about simple writing:

> Writing simply and clearly is not easy. Anne Tyler writes that 'it's hard to be simple, the hardest thing there is'. On the other hand, direct writing *feels* right. 'When I see a paragraph shrinking under my eyes like a strip of bacon in a skillet', Peter De Vries says, 'I know I'm on the right track'.
>
> Strong 1991

Prefer the familiar word

Use words that everyone knows. Don't use 'notion' when you mean 'idea'. Avoid 'pedestrian' when you mean boring. And so on. Most of us have words that we *enjoy* using. Be careful of them. A famous writer in the last century wrote that whenever he came upon a passage in his work that he particularly liked, he crossed it out. We can easily fool ourselves that we are writing everlasting prose. Mostly, we are not. Keep it simple. Or, as the Americans would have it: observe the KISS principle. Keep It Simple, Stupid. In a similar but different vein, Gillett offers the following advice on finding the 'right' words:

> The right words are those that are:
> concrete, rather than abstract
> short, rather than long

familiar, rather than unfamiliar
direct, rather than roundabout
economical, rather than flowery.

Gillett 1990

On the other hand, none of this means that you have to be *boring*.
It is important to continue to explore words and their meanings.
Seventy years ago, Dorothea Brande had this to say:

> Be on the alert to find appropriate words wherever you read,
> but before you use them be sure they are congruous when
> side by side with words of your own vocabulary. Combing a
> thesaurus for what an old professor of mine used to call,
> contemptuously, 'vivid verbs' will be far less useful than to
> find words in the midst of a living story; although a
> thesaurus is a good tool if it is used as it is meant to be.

Brande 1934

Avoid unnecessary words

Another straightforward one. Try to cut out the 'howevers' and the
'nevertheless'. Avoid qualifying adjectives with 'very' (as in: it is very
important that student social workers . . .). Especially avoid double
qualification ('very, very').

I have a soft spot for the word 'vital'. If I am not careful, I find
myself writing tired old sentences that start: 'It is vital that health
professionals . . .'. As you read through this book, notice how often I
use the word. Hopefully, you won't find it at all. Having
acknowledged my overuse of it, I have tried to prune it out. Try to do
this with your own favourites. Note, too, that with a word processor,
it is easy to seek out these 'favourites' and put in other, more varied,
words. The Search and Replace features help you to do this.

Put action in your verbs

Action gets people moving. Words like 'go' and 'move' keep people
reading. Try to make your writing active rather than passive. There is
still a tendency in the academic world for everything to be written in
the past tense. Try breaking that rule. Also, avoid clumsy locutions (!)
such as: 'The writer feels that . . .' or 'The current author
acknowledges that . . .'. It is better to write 'I think that . . .'. After
all, it must be clear that *you* are the writer or author. If not, who is?

Write like you talk

This is an important one but one that is easily ignored. The
statement itself is an example of 'writing like you talk'. More

grammatically, it should be 'write as you talk'. But who would *say* something like: 'I feel that it is of considerable importance that clients in the health profession are offered the provision of counselling'? No one. If you tend to write in this way, try clipping those sorts of sentence down like this: 'People should be offered counselling when they want it'. Much clearer. The test of whether or not you are observing this rule is to read out what you have written. If you would not say it, do not write it. This applies to both fiction and non-fiction.

This is, I appreciate, a contentious issue. Not everyone will want to write like they speak and nor will everyone want *others* to write like *they* speak. A lot will depend on the sort of language style that the writer adopts in everyday life. Clearly, the following would not be a very acceptable style of writing in an academic essay

> It's, like, Freud described the unconscious. He can't have been the first. After all, there must have been an unconscious before Freud arrived – but you get what I mean: he was the first, as far as we know, to put it all into words. He seemed to have known what he was on about, if you get my drift.

Claiborne (1990), in a study of the use of the English language, cites some examples of some particularly bad written material, from American sources:

- **A first-year college student**: 'It's obvious, in our modern world of today, there's a lot of impreciseness in expressing thoughts we have.'

- **A candidate for an MA at a large Midwestern university**: 'If you know the problems, the children are difficult to evaluate with.'

- **A doctor**: 'Symptomatology relative to impending or incipient onset of illness generally manifests itself initially via a marked chill, followed by a rapid rise of temperature to the 103 degree – 105 degree range is characteristically observed.'

- **A teacher (!) writing to a parent**: 'Scott is dropping in his studies he acts as if he don't Care. Scott want pass in his assignment at all, he had a poem to learn and he fell tu do it.'

- **A book review in the New Yorker**: 'If he were trying to pull himself together by hanging on to Esther's sanity, and she knew that and parlayed it, there would be come dynamics and edges.'

Claiborne 1990

What Gunning was suggesting, though, was that there is no need to use *complicated* language in writing. When we write, we often use a lot of padding that we do not use in speech. The 'read it out loud' principle described above is a good way of weeding out the superfluities.

Use terms your reader can picture

Try to use metaphors and illustrations that create pictures for the reader. Just because you are writing a report does not mean that you cannot 'illustrate' your writing in this way. Be careful, though. Make sure that you do not mix metaphors. This, apart from being grammatically wrong (which is not a big problem), causes all sorts of problems with imagery. My favourite mixed metaphor is one I heard a psychiatrist use: 'We all leaned over backwards to oil the wheels for this patient'. Oddly enough, this is a mixed metaphor that you *can* picture but the picture is a strange one.

On this sort of issue, avoid 'the screamer'. The screamer is the writing trade's name for the exclamation mark. If something is funny or ironic, the reader will notice. You don't have to rub their nose in it. If you do use an exclamation mark, only ever use one. Never use two or three!!! Keep multiple exclamation marks for reminder notes you leave yourself on the top of the TV to remember to pay the bills.

Tie in with your reader's experience

Illustrate what you write with small 'case studies' or illustrations from life. Invite the reader to think of her own examples of what you are talking about. At the same time, avoid rhetorical questions. It is irritating to read questions that seem to hang in the air without an answer. Isn't it?

Make full use of variety

If you can, use things to help your reader to keep awake. If you are writing an article for a journal, use checklists and boxed 'word illustrations'. This helps to break up large chunks of text. Look through any magazine that you have to hand. What you will find is that only the academic journals use continuous blocks of text. All others use variety to keep the reader interested. On the other hand, don't use these devices for their own sake. Make sure that they add to the reader's understanding of your writing.

Write to express not impress

This is the ultimate point. Your aim is not to show how clever you are. It should be to communicate your ideas to other people. This point seems to summarise all the other ones. Many students, when they start to write essays for diploma and degree courses, think that they have to try to imitate the worst sorts of academic writing. Perhaps they read journal papers in fairly dull journals. Perhaps some of their lecturers talk in that way. Whatever the reason, the point is to stop writing in that fashion. Write simply, clearly and use the obvious word rather than the more complicated one.

Reflective activity

Consider the following extract from a nursing book and think about whether or not it could have been written more clearly (you may even want to consider what it *means*):

> The ability to engage in self-care is also conceptualized as having form and content. Self-care agency is conceptualized as taking the form of a set of human abilities for deliberate action: the ability to attend to specific things (this includes the ability to exclude other things) and to understand their characteristics and the meaning of the characteristics; the ability to apprehend the need to change or regulate the things observed; the ability to acquire knowledge of appropriate courses of action for regulation; the ability to decide what to; and the ability to act to achieve change or regulation. The content of self-care agency derives from its proper object, meeting self-care requisites, whatever those requisites are at specific moments.
>
> Orem 1980

George Orwell, quoted in the *Economist Pocket Style Book* (Grimond 1986) offered a similar but different list of recommendations. Orwell's 'six elementary rules', in his 1946 book *Politics and the English Language*, were as follows. While they offer similar advice to Gunning's, they also highlight some other important stylistic issues:

1. Never use a *metaphor*, simile or other figure of speech which you are used to seeing in print
2. Never use a long word where a *short* word will do
3. If it is possible to cut out a word, always cut it out
4. Never use the passive where you can use the *active*
5. Never use a *foreign phrase*, a scientific word or a jargon word if you can think of an everyday English equivalent
6. Break any of these rules sooner than say anything outright barbarous.

Writing, then, should be fresh, straightforward and well constructed. There is no need to use difficult words, foreign phrases for effect or unnecessary jargon. In the next section, we explore jargon.

The use of jargon

Interestingly – and no doubt, correctly – almost any book you read about writing stresses the need for *simplicity*. The suggestion is usually that sentences and paragraphs should be short and that the simpler word should be preferred to the more complicated. And yet it is possible to pick up very many medical texts and find complicated, not to say impenetrable writing. Hudson (1978) in his book *The Jargon of the Professions* identifies the sorts of writers who are particularly at risk from using complicated and jargon-ridden writing. According to Hudson, they are:

- Those who are insecure and who feel they must do everything possible to make society feel that it needs their services
- Those who are ashamed of what they do and are driven to find suitable language with which to gild their activities
- Those who need big words, as they need big cars, to give them an extra ration of size
- Those who have nothing really to sell, and who need jargon in order to hoodwink the customers.

In these consumer-driven days, it is to be hoped that, in the health-care professions, no one is trying to 'hoodwink the customers'. Some health-care writers may, however, be tempted to hoodwink each other with complicated language and with wild abstractions.

On the other hand, there is also an 'up' side to jargon. In certain research papers and articles submitted to learned journals, a small amount of jargon may be used as a shorthand. If it is known that a piece of writing is going to be read by an audience of limited size and made up of like-minded professionals then it may be useful to use a certain amount of jargon. Clearly, it would be impractical to explain and define *every* term in these circumstances. The objection to jargon is when it is being used for the reasons discussed in the previous paragraphs.

Abstraction

Abstractions are popular. They are hard to refute and often lead to the writer sounding more clever than she really is – it also allows them to live in the clouds. Sir Ernest Gowers, in a classic book about clear writing, had this to say about the use of abstract words:

> Unfortunately the very vagueness of abstract words is one of the reasons for their popularity. To express one's thoughts

accurately is hard work, and to be precise is sometimes dangerous. We are tempted to prefer the safer obscurity of the abstract. It is the greatest vice of present-day writing.

Gowers 1962

And that was more than 40 years ago.

This is not to suggest that abstracts should *never* be discussed but, perhaps, to note that even abstract ideas should be grounded in reality. In practical professions such as the medical and paramedical professions, it would seem vital that ideas about those professions link very much with 'real life'. Sadly, a reading of some of the health-care journals does not always bear out this direct relationship.

Complicated writing is sometimes encouraged by some academics' persistence in recommending the 'third person' as the only appropriate tense in academic writing. It has become a cliché in education that, for some reason, students completing courses should always avoid 'I' or 'we' in their writing. Instead, they should offer peculiar locutions such as 'in the present writer's view' or 'in the opinion of this author'. Who, if not 'I', is writing these words?

Third person

The injunction to use the 'third person' is based on the fallacy that 'this is how academics write'. Kirkman (1992) in a survey of 81 academic journals from a wide range of disciplines – and all peer-reviewed – found that only 7 did not contain papers in which 'I', 'we' or 'our' featured. Put the other way, 74 academic journals allowed the use of these. Included in the list that did allow this usage was perhaps the most prestigious journal of all – *Nature*. None of this means that papers and articles have to be a litany of 'I's but just to acknowledge that if it is simpler to say 'I' then it is probably better.

Following Gunning (1968), there is a very simple test to see whether or not your writing is clear and simple. You read it out loud. If you find yourself thinking 'I would never *say* that', then the writing can probably be rephrased. After all, in speech – as we have noted – we would not be allowed to get away with being too complicated. In speech, we are likely to be challenged. Our writing, then, should imitate our speech. We should seek the transparent, the clear and the uncomplicated. Grammar – as Gowers was at pains to point out – should be a guide to writing, not an immutable law.

This is not to say that nothing written should ever be complex. It is quite possible to convey complex ideas clearly. Unfortunately, too

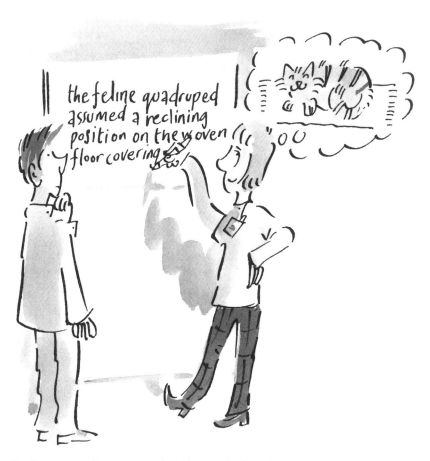

Don't over-complicate your writing. Keep it simple and clear.

often, it is the person who has little that is complex to say who wraps her ideas up in language (Kirkman 1992). This, then, is not a call for reducing everything to its lowest common denominator – far from it. It is a call for clear writing.

In the end, of course, words and meanings are slippery. Just as we think we have written something that is ambiguous, someone else will come along and ask us what we mean. The production of a completely clear piece of writing is probably something out of reach. On the other hand, an examination of how we communicate orally gives us a clue to how we understand other people. Orally, we tend to work in approximations. We think we understand the other person and work on the basis that we have until the other person indicates otherwise. With writing, of course, there is no 'second chance' – the author is no longer around to explain any mistakes nor to clarify meanings. However, most of us don't read every word in a book, nor do we work through passages a word at a time. Instead, we build up an impression of what the writer means. Indeed, some fiction depends on this process. This is probably the best we can hope for – even in non-fiction. We should not, though, make the job any more difficult than it is already. Our aim, I maintain, is to write as clearly as we can and that almost always means simply. We all work with two vocabularies: an active one (the one we use in everyday life) and a passive one (which contains words we understand but don't use very often).

Note, that the passive vocabulary often contains more than its fair share of abstract terms and may contain many 'approximations'. By 'approximations' I mean those words about which we have an idea of their meaning but would be hard pushed to pin it down. What, for example, do the words 'phenomenology', 'positivism', 'paradigm' and 'humanism' really mean? My guess is that lots of different people would give you lots of different definitions – and many would claim to be right. Accessing the active vocabulary is likely to make both you and the reader more inclined to read on than if you are always tugging at your own and the reader's passive vocabulary.

The psychologist David Canter makes an interesting observation about the changing nature of words and – in particular – about the turning of nouns into verbs. Writing about the jargon attached to the psychology of crime, he writes:

> The term 'offender profiling' has stuck; yet another example of the admirably creative but infuriatingly confusing American reinvention of English words and phrases. Often the key to these word inventions is to take a noun in common use, preferably a noun that is reasonably abstract and is therefore used to describe a relatively complex phenomenon, such as 'police', 'priority' or 'interface', and to turn these into verbs where none existed before. A rather unclear notion emerges, rich in resonance: 'to police', 'to prioritize', 'to interface'. Now with skilled prestidigitation the verb can creep back in as a noun, but now it is describing a process: 'policing', 'prioritizing' 'interfacing'. Because of its roots in a reasonably specific well-known noun the impression is created that a distinct process exists that can be cut and dried and sold by the pound.
>
> Canter 1994

Over to you

Can you think of any other nouns which have undergone a similar transformation recently and have become verbs?

On the other hand, you may want to take Canter to task for using words like 'prestidigitation'.

Avoid 'sic'

The word 'sic' is sometimes put in brackets after a direct quotation from someone else's work. It is there to indicate that the current writer acknowledges that the passage is not quite right, grammatically or in terms of spelling or structure. What it can convey is something like this:

> I realise, of course, that this is not how you or I would write but I am clever enough to bring to your notice that I have spotted the writer's error. Like you, I would not make the same mistake in my own writing. In future, be cautious about everything this writer has to say. She might make similar mistakes again. She is not very reliable: keep her work at arm's length.

In other words, the use of 'sic' can sound smug. It is best avoided if at all possible. There are times when you need to indicate that an unusual form of words was used. If you are writing up a research report that calls for direct quotations from interviews, then you need to use the respondent's own words. All you have to do, here, is to acknowledge, at an early stage in your report that you are offering direct quotations. You don't have to pepper your report with 'sic'. An appropriate word if ever there was one.

Keeping a journal

Consider keeping a writing journal. Many people start writing a diary, fill it in for a few days or weeks and then abandon it. Call yours a journal and keep on filling it in. Buy a large spiral or hardbound notebook. Put a label on the front and then use the following headings to organise your entries:

- New ideas for writing
- Longer term goals for research or books

- Quotations (including full reference and page number)
- New references
- Notes about self (Keep a note of your productivity versus your mood. Some people write better when they are slightly miserable. Writing can be cathartic.)
- Writing completed. It is useful for your CV to have a running tally of the completed pieces of written work. This is particularly true if you have articles published in journals or magazines.

Carry the journal with you at all times, if you can. Keep it by your bed and don't be afraid of jotting down ideas in the middle of the night. It you don't jot them down then, the ideas will often be gone by the morning.

Every so often, perhaps once a month, read through your journal. Pull out the references and put them in your bibliographical database. See whether or not you want to pursue the ideas for articles and file away your new quotations. Sometimes, the quotations can be put in the references database.

Keep this sort of journal for at least six months. After that, it tends to become something of a habit. It is certainly a more reliable way of keeping track of your thoughts and ideas than jotting them down on the backs of envelopes. Even if writing on the backs of envelopes seems rather more romantic.

Take some time in choosing the sort of book that you will use for your journal. This sort of hunting down is not only pleasurable in itself but it helps to reinforce the idea that you are serious about keeping the journal. Write for yourself but ponder this thought from a friend of mine in the book trade. He feels that *all* writing is biographical and a form of exhibitionism.

Reflective activity

Consider your own views on the thought that all writing is biographical, and reread something that you have written. To what degree does that writing contain a part of you?

Also, consider *why* you write. I have suggested that writing may be cathartic. That is to say that it may be one way of our dealing with hidden conflicts and emotional stress. I don't want to be too psychological about all this. It is easy to dream up theories about why people do or don't do various things. Often, such theories are fairly spurious. It does seem to be true, however, that some forms of writing can be compulsive. Malcolm Bradbury has warned of how easy it can be to 'write yourself to death'. Hopefully, not too many of us do this. It is interesting, though, to ponder on one's motives for writing. Not for long, though. Much more important is the production of readable and hopefully saleable copy.

Top tips

Write simply and clearly:
- Avoid unnecessary jargon
- Use short sentences and short paragraphs
- Spell check your work carefully.

Writing habits

I find it useful to be slightly ritualistic about writing. I try to write every day and I tend to start writing at much the same time. Brande, writing of the need to write regularly and to order, suggests the following:

> After you have dressed, sit down for a moment by yourself and go over the day before you. Usually you can tell accurately enough what its demands and opportunities will be; roughly, at the least, you can sketch out for yourself enough of your program to know what you when you will have a few moments to yourself. It need not be very long; fifteen minutes will do nicely. . . . Decide for yourself when you will take that time for writing; for you are going to write in it. . . . Now this is very important, and can hardly be emphasized too strongly: *you have decided to write at four o'clock, and at four o'clock write you must! No excuses can be given.*
>
> Brande 1934

First, I read through what I finished the evening before and then I carry on. I don't edit anything until I have finished the whole of a project and I try not to keep crossing out. I feel that it is important to develop a sense of flow. Although it has been said that what is easy to produce is likely to make easy reading, I feel that the opposite can also be true. If you slave for hours over every word you can end up with pages of stilted and difficult to read text. This is the odd paradox: you have to be careful about what you write but not so careful that it interferes with what you want to say.

If you want to check how readable your work is, consider investing in one of the Shareware programs that will 'read' and comment on your work. Usually, such programs offer you a 'FOG rating' index – a measure of how readable your work is (most of the larger word-processing programs also have a feature that will do this for you). As a rule, it is short sentences and simple words that win the day in the readability stakes. When you string together lengthy prose, you lose your reader. If necessary, go back and break up sentences with full stops. I often find this to be necessary. I have a habit of dividing sentences with colons. I can nearly always go back and replace the colon with a full stop. Colons, semi-colons and other such 'complicated' punctuation should be used sparingly.

Style

This is the most difficult thing of all to define. Style is not content. It refers to the way in which words are put together. Kirkman (1992) defines it like this:

> Style in writing is concerned with choice. Every writer has available the enormous resources of a whole language. English presents a particularly large range of choices of individual words, and of combinations of words into small and large 'structures' – idioms, phrases, clauses, sentences, paragraphs, sections, chapters. The choices we make create the 'style', which is a term covering balance, emphasis and tone.
>
> Kirkman 1992

Like other sorts of reading, it is worth learning to read for style. This is easier with fiction than with non-fiction. Style is, however, present in non-fiction even if it is almost buried by the content. Too often, the style in non-fiction slips by us because we are caught up with the content. On the other hand, we do notice the style in that we readily dismiss that book as 'bad' and this one as 'easy to read'. The hardest thing of all is to begin to notice your own style. There is something paradoxical here. If you work at developing a style, you are likely to lose it. You begin to turn out pieces that are self-conscious.

Top tips

Forget your own style but work away at getting the following things in order:

- Sentence construction
- Paragraph construction
- Use of new metaphors
- Clear use of description
- Interesting reporting of research
- Ability to inspire the reader
- Enough 'padding' between hard facts to keep the reader reading.

This last point may not be completely obvious. We cannot keep throwing fact after fact at the reader. In between chunks of facts, we need to have a little relief. This can come as criticism or commentary on what has gone before. Notice how other writers use this. Do not be tempted to pare down your style of writing so much that you leave out any sort of padding. On the other hand, be wary of page filling for the sake of it. Lecturers and tutors who have to mark essays will be very aware of students' attempts at such page filling. A good example of this is the following:

> All health professionals, almost by definition, have to care. The whole process of caring is important in that it shows how a relationship between one person and another can develop in very meaningful ways. If we do not care we cannot be seen as real professionals nor can we be seen as true carers. Most health-care workers prefer to see their work as having professional elements to it. Perhaps the caring aspect is the most important element of all. The question remains, however, how do we define care and what research has been done on the topic? These questions and many others are the subject of this essay. Essentially, it is vital that we fully appreciate the metaparadigm that lies behind the philosophy of care that the health professional is offering *vis à vis* the client.

In offering advice to sub-editors, Jill Baker (1987) discusses the following basic rules of style:

- Rewrite long sentences
- Replace pompous or polysyllabic words with simpler ones

- Make sure that the author's sentence construction is clear
- Omit unnecessary adjectives and omit qualifications such as 'very'
- Ensure that words are used precisely
- Make sure that verbs are active
- Make sure that the author uses metaphors correctly and sparingly
- Replace jargon with a phrase in everyday use.

Finally, you must *care* about what you write. Writing is rarely a simple, mechanical process. When it is, it is usually obvious to the reader. Strong (1991) sums this up as follows:

> Caring about what you write is the starting point. If *you* don't care about what you say and how you say it, why should anyone else? An indifferent attitude almost guarantees that no one will take you seriously. Communication in writing is like any human relationship: Nothing important or interesting happens unless you really care.
>
> Strong 1991

Punctuation

Like it or not, you need to get punctuation right. This is especially true if you are submitting work for examination or assessment. If you are sending in a manuscript for publication, the chances are that a sub-editor will help to modify your punctuation if it is wrong. On the other hand, you are less likely to have your work accepted for publication if your punctuation is obviously poorly used. It is worth considering Carey's comments on the use of punctuation:

> Stops should be used as sparingly as sense will permit: but in so far as they are needed for an immediate grasp of the sense or for the avoidance of any possible ambiguity, or occasionally to relieve a very lengthy passage, they should be used as freely as need be. The best punctuation is that of which the reader is least conscious; for when punctuation, or the lack of it, obtrudes itself, it is usually because it offends.
>
> Carey 1976

Here are some general pointers about punctuating.

- **Full stop (.)** Used at ends of sentences. Called a 'period' in North America. As in: 'I'm broke. Period.'
- **Comma (,)**: Used between phrases, within sentences and in lists – as in 'He was tall, dark and extremely ugly' or 'We sent them dates, prunes and pineapples.'
- **Semi-colon (;)**: Used, in long sentences, to break up sections. It is often better to insert a full stop rather than use a semi-colon. Examples: 'She walked on her hands as part of the circus performance; sometimes she stood in for one of the clowns.' or 'She walked on her hands as part of the circus performance. Sometimes she stood in for one of the clowns.'
- **Colon (:)**: Used at the end of one phrase and the beginning of another, for emphasis or as the introduction to a list. Examples: 'The room was almost full: it would have been difficult to pack in any more people.' 'When you go on holiday, you may want to consider taking the following: your passport, money, something to read.'
- **Hyphen or dash (-)** Used to 'insert a phrase into a sentence, almost as an 'aside'. Examples: 'Fresh fish is a good buy – as are sausages – for the person who wants a cheap meal'. Also used to indicate a break in a word at the end of a line in a book.
- **Inverted commas (')** Used around speech and, sparingly, to highlight a word or phrase, sometimes with irony. Not to be overused as a means of emphasis. For example: 'Don't call me that!' she said, obviously angry. He was 'gutted' by the response he got following the distribution of the questionnaires.
- **Exclamation mark (!)** Used – and overused – as a form of exclamation or emphasis. Sometimes used to indicate that a sentence is meant to be funny. If it is, it should stand up for itself, without the exclamation mark. If in doubt, do not use an exclamation mark.

- If in doubt, keep punctuation simple
- Use full stops rather than colons and semi-colons to break up text
- Instead of using lots of commas, put in a full stop
- Begin to notice how other people use punctuation. Start, if you like, by looking at the way it is used in this book.

Practise writing

There are certain exercises that you can do to improve your writing. First, try the process know as 'free writing'. Get up every morning and sit down at the computer. Then begin to type. Type anything that comes into your head. At first, do not attempt to disallow anything that comes to mind. The aim is to get as much writing done in the shortest time possible. Start by doing this for 2 minutes and build up to doing it for 10 minutes. As you get better at it, begin to pay attention to the form and content of the writing. Do not go to the keyboard with a specific idea in mind but gradually, as ideas come to you, begin to quickly work them into shape. Do all this without prior planning and without doing an outline for what you are writing. Here is an example of free writing:

```
It's cold in here and I have to write about groups. The
important thing about groups is facilitation. Probably.
Possibly. Perhaps the most important thing about groups
is being in one. Think of groups that I have been in.
Where do I start? Groups from schooldays: classes, cubs,
scouts and so on. Groups from teenage years: friends,
parties. Professional groups. Not that I belong to any at
the moment. Should I join one? Why do people join groups?
Sometimes, of course, they have no choice. Primary and
secondary groups: note the differences. Is there anyone
out there who does not belong to some group or other? I
doubt it. Even the ones that weren't in groups would be
members of a group called 'people who don't live in
groups'. What a thought: no escape.
```

This exercise is one of the best ones for dealing with writers' block and it is also excellent for encouraging you to work quickly. Later on (or even sooner) you may be asked to write a column for a magazine in your profession. If you do that, you will have to write quickly. Often, you will be asked for about 1000 words by the end of the week. You have no choice, then. You have to write quickly. Keep this exercise going for a few weeks or consider keeping it going all the time. John Braine, the author, found this activity a particular useful one for helping him to work quickly and accurately.

✍ *Over to you*

Another activity consists of editing a passage of writing. Read through the passage in Figure 1.1 and consider how you could improve it. Pay particular attention to the following points:

- Sentence and paragraph construction
- Phrasing
- Use of words
- Any unnecessary words of phrases
- The flow of the piece.

The term 'health professional' covers a multitude of sins: health professionals can range from occupational therapists, to doctors and from nurses to other sorts of health care workers, although not everyone likes that label. What distinguishes health care professionals from other sorts of health care workers? This is an important question and one that demands to be answered soon if we are to offer a viable and healthy service to patients, clients, residents and other consumers of care. Perhaps it is the word 'professional'. The word 'professional' has many connotations and many meanings. It means different things to different people. To some it means one thing and to others it means something else. In this paper, I plan to consider the word 'professional' and try to identify what it means as it relates to the health professions. The term 'professional' is widely used to describe widely differing sorts of occupations and jobs. For example, it is possible to talk about 'professional footballers' but no one would, normally, compare professional footballers to, say, lawyers who are also professionals but different sorts of professionals. Some writers have attempted to identify the sorts of criteria that can be used to distinguish professionals from non-professionals and these methods will be discussed in the next few paragraphs. What is important from the point of view of the health care professional is also to look at the literature on health care and trace the history of those workers to the present day in which the idea of professionalisation has become an important issue.

Figure 1.1 *Text to edit*

As you work through this activity, consider the style of the piece. Did you enjoy reading it? Was it lively? Did it have zest? Did you want to read more? If not, consider why not. Make the changes that you would make if you were being asked to publish the piece in a newspaper or magazine. Your task is to make the passage readable and interesting. As you do this, notice to what degree your own writing problems are contained in the passage. Do you fall into the traps that this writer did or are your shortcomings different ones?

Part of the process of becoming an effective writer is to know something about your own style of writing. It is often possible to see it reflected in the writings of others. That is why it is useful to be asked to be a reviewer for a journal or magazine. You are unlikely to be paid for the task but it will quickly teach you what editors do and do not accept as suitable copy for publication.

> ### Over to you
>
> Read a variety of health-care journals and compare their styles. Some will make full use of subheadings (often of the single-word variety). These tend to be used to break up solid blocks of text. The more academic journals presumably assume that their readers have more staying power. They use fewer headings and the headings tend to be more descriptive and accurate. Few journals or magazines have no subheadings at all. Notice, too, how paragraphs are laid out in magazines and journals. Because most are printed in double columns, editors tend to prefer short paragraphs. In double-column layout, these are easier to read. Try to spot exceptions to this rule. Sometimes, an editor of an academic journal will not do substantial editing of a particular paper. Often, such papers have longer paragraphs than usual. As ever, the nearer you can get your own work to the publishable standard, the better it is likely to be. It is quite easy to learn the basics of layout.

Simplicity and structure

These remain the keywords. All the best writing is simple in style. All the best writing (except, perhaps, the '**stream of consciousness**' writers like James Joyce and Virginia Woolf – but we are not in their league) is structured. A simple writing style is not always easy to achieve. It can be made easier, though, if you try to avoid 'fillers' such as the following:

- There is a sense in which . . .
- However . . .
- It is the writer's view that . . .
- It is sometimes the case that . . .
- The writer would like to forward the view that . . .
- We have to consider this over and against the other view that . . . .

All of these hide the message. Sometimes academics use them to try to hedge their bets. It is as if they are saying to the reader: 'I know there are other points of views and this may not be the right one and that there are a whole range of other things that could be said here but . . .'. In the end, we have to be prepared to stick to

Keywords

Stream of consciousness
A method of writing in which thoughts, reactions and ideas are written without interruption by objective description or dialogue

what we want to say and say it. It really is as simple as that. Mostly we are not writing philosophy so we don't have to ponder over every nuance of meaning and possibility. Take some risks. Declare what you want to say without the wrapping. But . . . keep it structured.

Paragraphs

A paragraph is a collection of sentences that deals with one united topic. Paragraphs help the reader to follow different parts of an argument. Each sentence within a paragraph needs to connect coherently with the others. A well-built paragraph is easy to follow and links well to the paragraph before and after it. The final sentence has a function, in that it forms the starting point for the next paragraph. Paragraphs that are well constructed will begin by linking back to the previous paragraph.

👉 *Over to you*

Here are two paragraphs from a student's assignment. Read these, and decide what linking sentence(s) you would use to help this part of the essay to flow.

A number of staff contribute to the clinical learning environment for student nurses. Despite this, the support and quality of teaching provided for student nurses continues to be an area for concern (Birchenall 2001). Mentors play a vital role, but many of these nurses are not clear about what is encompassed in a mentorship role (Neary 1997). This lack of clarity suggests that mentors are often inadequately prepared for their role. Some mentors see the support of student nurses as fundamental to their job, while others view this as an additional responsibility (Pulsford *et al.* 2002). For most mentors, getting through the working day is the first priority, giving quality of care the second, and supporting students the third (ENB 2000).

Students perceived 'poor' teachers as those who were unapproachable, lacking in empathy and providing little support or encouragement (Morgan & Knox 1987). In contrast, Hanson & Smith (1996) found that small acts or episodes where a teacher paid attention to the student and helped them to believe in their ability to be a nurse were highly valued caring interactions. It helps if in a clinical link role capacity, nurse teachers undertake prearranged visits at least twice per month with all of the students allocated to the clinical area (Wills 1997). Support strategies need to be in place in clinical areas to allow students to express their views, opinions and feelings in an atmosphere of psychological safety (Quinn 2000).

Counting words

A professional writer counts words. She has to. Most professionals are paid according to the number of words they write. Most professionals, too, are told the limit of the words they can write. This book, for example, should be about 75,000–85,000 words in length. If I wrote 120,000 words, the editor would probably complain and might send the manuscript back. If I wrote 200,000 words, she certainly would. If, on the other hand, I sent in a manuscript of 35,000 words, she would send that back too. There is little margin for negotiation once limits have been set. This is also true for essays, dissertations and projects. Find out the limit and then work to it but don't go over it. Also, the discipline of working to a set number of words can tighten up your style. Prefer to work to a word limit and see the development of your writing. You can say a lot in 1,000 words and a lot in 100,000.

The real basics

Michael Larson (1986) offers the following checklist for prospective writers. His list (which includes an essential American book about writing) is appropriate to all would-be writers in the health professions. He maintains that all writers should have:

- Something to say
- The compulsive need to say it
- Talent: the gift for turning ideas into words, characters and the situations and knowing when they are right
- Discipline
- Persistence
- Faith in your work
- Trust in your instincts
- Patience with your talents and others' appreciation of it
- Reading
- The *Elements of Style* by William Strunk Jr and E.B. White
- The need to grow as a writer and the experience with art and life to do so.

Larson 1986

The next book to read is Strunk and White.

> ## ꞦꞦꞦꞦꞦRapid recap
>
> Check your progress so far by working through each of the following questions.
>
> 1. List three things which help the presentation of your writing.
> 2. List four ways to improve your writing style.
> 3. When might you see the use of 'sic'?
>
> If you have difficulty with more than one of the questions, read through the section again to refresh your understanding before moving on.

References

Baker, J. (1987) *Copy Prep*. Blueprint, London.

Bennett, A. (1994) *Writing Home*. Faber & Faber, London.

Brande, D. (1934) *Becoming a Writer*. Harcourt Brace, New York.

Canter, D. (1994) *Criminal Shadows*. Harper/Collins, London.

Carey, G.V. (1976) *Mind the Stop*. Penguin, Harmondsworth.

Claiborne, R. (1990) *The Life and Times of the English Language: The history of our marvellous native tongue*. Bloomsbury, London.

Docherty, T. (ed.) (1993) *Postmodernism: A reader*. Harvester Wheatsheaf, New York.

Gillett, H. (1990) *Study Skills: A guide for health care professionals*. Distance Learning Centre, South Bank Polytechnic, London.

Gowers, E. (1962) *The Complete Plain Words*. Penguin, Harmondsworth.

Grimond, J. (1986) *The Economist Pocket Style Book*. The Economist, London.

Gunning, R. (1968) *The Technique of Clear Writing*, 2nd edn. McGraw-Hill, London.

Hudson, K. (1978) *The Jargon of the Professions*. Macmillan, London.

Kirkman, J. (1992) *Good Style: Writing for science and technology*. E. & F.N. Spon, London.

Larson, M. 1986 *Literary Agents: How to get and work with the right one for you*. Writer's Digest Books, Cincinnati, OH.

Orem, D. (1980) *Nursing: Concepts of practice*, 2nd edn. McGraw-Hill, New York.

Strong, W. (1991) *Writing Incisively: Do-it-yourself prose surgery*. McGraw-Hill, New York.

Strunk, W. and White, E.B. (1999) *The Elements of Style*, 2nd edn. Macmillan, New York.

2

Equipment and environment

The bookful blockhead, ignorantly read,
With loads of learned lumber in his head.
Alexander Pope

Most of the people I know seem to like buying stationery. There is something attractive about the pads and files you find in the shops. This chapter identifies some of the equipment you may want to consider if you are going to write. It will be a short chapter. These days, the basic and most important item of equipment is the computer. If you want to write and you do not have one, buy one. It will change the way you write, conclusively.

Where to write

I have been looking at a book about studying. It goes into great detail about how you should set aside a room that is reserved for your books and files and in which you quietly gather your thoughts and do your work. Who can afford this sort of extra-room-luxury? Most of us are struggling to find space in the houses that we already have.

My advice is simply this. Find out how you work best. Then, as long as it continues to work, work in that way. I, for example, sit in a corner of the dining room, tapping away at the keys of my computer while, in the adjoining living room, my family sit and watch TV, shout at each other and do all the things that families always do. A large dog and two cats sometimes come and worry me but generally I am left alone. If I want to, I can get up and wander into the kitchen to make coffee. Sometimes it is made for me. I can also get up and go and watch the 10 o'clock news when it comes on. It is not a good idea to sit in front of a computer screen for hours on end. Watching another screen at least gets you away from the smaller one for a few minutes. Also, it allows you to stretch and it saves you from getting repetitive strain injury from prolonged periods at the keyboard.

I have a pile of books on the floor next to me that I use while I am writing. At the end of a session (if I am in the right mood), I put them all away in bookshelves. Otherwise, I am almost ashamed to write, they stay where they are, until I move them another day or someone else clears them away.

This is the way that I work. It may not suit you. I find that I don't particularly like the cloistered life and don't work well in quiet places. On the other hand, I am not someone who works with a radio or personal stereo on. Instead, I prefer a fairly 'normal' domestic background. It tends to help me keep my feet on the ground and I hope that this means that my writing is more straightforward. All this applies to any sort of writing project. I adopt the same style of working if I am writing up a research report and if I am writing a short article or a book. As I say, it works for me. What works for you?

Reflective activity

Consider the following places to work. Which would be ideal for you?
- In a quiet office of your own
- In a public library
- In the living room with the television on
- In your bedroom
- Outside
- In a hotel room
- In an office at work.

Now consider where you actually work. I suspect that most of us have to compromise to some degree about our writing environment. Could you make yours better?

By way of example, the American writer, William Strong describes how he works at making initial drafts of written work:

> For me, drafting often works in places like McDonald's where nobody hassles you, the coffee refills are free, and there's a low level of background noise. I prefer pens with laser-like tips. I have an aversion to slick, clay-coated paper and a fondness for cheap note pads, especially soft yellow ones. How about you?
>
> Strong 1991

Theory into practice

Find out if there is quiet space in your university department. Also, make full use of the learning resource centre, where computers may contain programs and files of information that will be useful to your clinical practice.

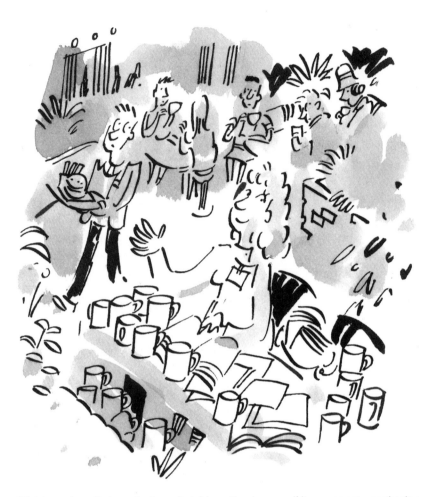

Stick to a place that you feel comfortable writing in, even if it may seem unorthodox.

Basic equipment

Certain basic things do seem to count as essentials. While the description above may sound a little rough and ready, my corner of the dining room is fairly well equipped. I consider that the following are essentials:

- A desk or table
- A computer
- A supply of lined pads
- A supply of computer paper, either continuous (if you use a dot matrix printer) or single sheets (if you use an ink jet or laser printer)

- A pot containing plenty of pens and pencils. I find I have to buy new supplies of these regularly as my family help themselves fairly freely. I am also aware that it took me months to find the right sort of pot to put them in. I finally tracked it down in Brittany
- A ruler, compass and other drawing implements (for drawing diagrams). If you use a computer well, you may be able to use it for your diagrams
- Bookshelves
- A filing cabinet (by no means essential to everyone but important if you have a tidy mind and like a tidy home)
- Sellotape on a heavy dispenser so that it stays put when you pull the tape
- A stapler and a large supply of staples
- Paperclips (but keep these away from your printer and from your computer keyboard)
- A clipboard for holding papers while you type at the keyboard
- A disk box for your floppy disks. It cannot be stated too clearly that you *must* back-up your computer work as you go. Hard disks in computers fail. If they fail and you have not backed up your work, you have lost it
- Sticky Post-it pads. These are vital for jotting down notes and for keeping a running tally of the number of words that you have written if you are working on a larger project. I like to write a new one at the end of each working session and to leave the old ones in place. In this way, the sheer volume of Post-its tells me how near I am to finishing the project
- A comfortable chair. Some of the older How To Study books describe the importance of a stoic approach to seating. I would sit in an armchair to work if I could fit one into my work setting. Be comfortable as you work. I can find no place for a straight-backed chair. If you need to be kept awake while you work, you have probably been working too long anyway.

If you intend to carry on writing, you will have to think carefully about bookshelves. We have about five large bookshelves in our house and all of them are full. As a result, we have books piled up everywhere. Sod's law dictates that the book you want is never one that is in a bookshelf. Also, such an arrangement does not endear you to libraries. It is always library books that fall down the backs of piles or lie, spine facing away, at the bottom of a pile of other books. Try to keep library books in their own pile. In this way, you know where to find them and always have them to hand when the reminder notices start coming through the letter box.

Also, spend some time choosing the desk and chair that you will sit at as you work. There are a variety of purpose-built computer tables available if you are going to work with a computer (and I hope that you are, if you are serious about writing). Such tables can be bulky affairs or they can be economical of space to the point where each item of your equipment is piled one on top of the other in a tidy, if not particularly aesthetically pleasing tower.

Remember that you have to *live* with the furniture that you buy. While it should be functional, I believe that you should also feel comfortable at it. Be particularly wary of computer desks that have pull-out keyboard holders. In my experience, these tend to be set at a very low level. If you are happy to sit in a low chair, buy one. If not, look for something else. Make sure that your seat is comfortable. Some books about writing tend to take a Spartan approach to seating and suggest that the best work can only be done in a straight-backed chair. The chair that is best for you is one that you are comfortable in. Swivel chairs are widely available but tend not to be very supportive of the back. Some favour 'posture' seating that encourages you to 'kneel' in front of your working surface. These are better for your back and shoulders but try one out before you buy one. Not everyone can cope with sitting in a kneeling position for very long.

> **Key points | Top tips**
>
> - Develop a habit for working: same place, same equipment
> - Don't work for hours on end: take frequent breaks
> - *Do* work! Don't find other activities to fill the time and to distract you from writing.

There is one other piece of equipment that may be useful, depending on the way you write, and that is a dictating machine. Clearly, they were designed for use by those who do not use computers themselves but have someone else type out their work. They are, however, very useful for make notes and writing memos on the move. Ideas for essays, papers and articles can all be 'jotted down' by simply speaking into a dictating machine. They take a little getting used to and not everyone can make the shift from writing on paper or on a computer to speaking into a machine. They are, however, remarkably cheap and many are now 'voice-activated': they turn themselves on when you speak into them.

Those who *do* have other people who can type up their work may want to use a dictating machine for writing substantial documents. It is possible to dictate the whole of an essay, project, article or even a book. This is *definitely* not everyone's favourite way of working and to do it properly takes a lot of new learning. Dictation was not, for instance, P.G. Wodehouse's preferred way of working. Although he was writing of the problems of dictating to another person, the problem that he describes below apply just as much to dictating into a machine:

> Not that I ever thought of dictating [this book] to a stenographer. How anybody can compose a story by word of mouth, face to face with a bored looking secretary with a notebook is more than I can imagine. Yet many authors think nothing of saying 'Ready, Miss Spelvin? Take dictation. Quote No comma Lord Jasper Murgatroyd comma close quote said no better make it hissed Evangeline comma quote I would not marry you if you were the last man on earth close quote period Quote Well comma, I'm not that last man on earth comma so the point does not arise comma close quote replied Lord Jasper comma twirling his moustache cynically period. And so the long day wore on.
>
> If I started to do that sort of thing I should be feeling all the time that the girl was saying to herself as she took it down, 'Well, comma this beats me period How comma with homes for the feeble minded touting for customers on every side comma has a fathead like this Wodehouse succeeded in remaining at large all these years mark of interrogation.
>
> Wodehouse 1934

It isn't, of course, quite as complicated as this but you do have to learn to cast sentences and then to *say* 'full stop' at the end of each of them. Once learned, the process works quite well.

The rhythm of writing

Just as there are no hard and fast rules about environment, nor are there such rules about the way in which you work. I tend to write best of all late at night. I do not enjoy writing in the morning, so I tend to avoid it. On the other hand, I am not too sensitive about all this. If I have to write to a deadline, I write at any time of the day.

On the other hand, try to establish a rhythm to your work. It is often a good idea to get warmed up a little by doing various 'domestic' tasks before you settle down to real writing. You can, for instance, back up some files from your hard disk to floppies. You can sort out your reference cards of your files. Do treat this as 'warming up', though and not as work itself. The work really starts when you begin to write. If you have a block of some sort, type *anything* on to the screen to get you started. Alternatively, write the word 'the' at the top of the screen and you will have started. Don't feel that you have to write consecutively. I have explained, elsewhere in this book, that – in longer projects – it is often best to start with a chapter or a section that you will enjoy writing and to leave the trickier parts until you have really got into your stride.

If you can, write every day. Don't be a slave to this rule and if you cannot stand the thought of writing on a particular day, don't worry. You are unlikely to lose the ability to write. I am frequently surprised by how many writers complicate the writing process by setting up all sorts of apparent 'rules' about writing. There are none. Find out what suits you best and stick to it. When it stops working, change what you do. If this is a rule, it is an important one. Keep working while what you do is effective. When it ceases to be effective, do something else. It is a basic precept in psychotherapy that the last thing a neurotic person wants to do is to change. They want their symptoms to go away but they do not want to change themselves. Some writers and academics are like this. They want to become better writers but stick, stolidly, to one style of working. Try new things. Do it differently. Then, when it begins to fall into place, stick to the process. The late Derek Jarman, the film director, once wrote that 'if you are not a perfectionist, you can get a lot done'. I have found this to be a particularly useful aphorism. You don't have to be a perfectionist. Do the best you can and then accept what you have done. Do not aim at perfection: life is far too short.

₨₨₨₨₨**Rapid recap**

Check your progress so far by working through the following question.

1. What are the most important pieces of basic equipment when doing a significant amount of writing?

If you have difficulty with this question, read through the section again to refresh your understanding before moving on.

References

Strong, W. (1991) *Writing Incisively: Do-it-yourself prose surgery*. McGraw-Hill, New York.

Wodehouse, P.G. (1934) *Thank You Jeeves*. In: *The Jeeves Omnibus*. Hutchinson, London.

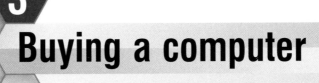

3

Buying a computer

Learning outcomes

By the end of this chapter you should be able to:

- Describe the differences between the types of computer available and their components

- Recognise some of the software packages available and their purposes

- Appreciate the importance of buying anti-virus software.

That's not writing, that's typing.

Truman Capote [of Jack Kerouac]

The point of this chapter is to identify some of the things that you will need to bear in mind if you are thinking of buying a computer to write with. And you should. There is still a lot of fear surrounding computers. Those who are not frightened by them sometimes take a superstitious view: 'I couldn't write straight into one' or 'it's not the same as writing on a pad of paper.' Of course it's not. It's much better. The big plus about writing with a computer is that you never have to rewrite. With a computer, you can bash out your draft, in any form you like. Then you can go slowly through the rushed draft and rescue the best bits. You can change a few words here, move a paragraph there. What you never have to do is start again, with a blank page, and write the whole thing again. That seems to me to be a considerable advantage.

Perhaps you take the view that you are too old to take up computing. Certainly, younger people work almost automatically with them. My teenage son taught me almost all I know about computers and computing. I have used a computer to write most of my books and papers and also used one to write course brochures, handouts, adverts, letters and so forth. I keep all my bibliographical references on a computer and I can quickly fish out exactly the reference I need, as I am writing. That means that I no longer have to filter through boxes of cards. A considerable time saver.

I am still surprised by what computers can do and how much time and effort they can save in the writing process. So: don't skip this chapter if you don't have a computer. Don't skip it if you do: there will be things here that you can use. For buying a computer for writing is slightly different from buying a computer as a games machine or as a general purpose household gadget.

Incidentally, it is not really necessary to know how a computer works in order to use one. I find it useful to think of them as the behavioural psychologists used to think of people. They tended to talk about the 'black box' approach to people: there were inputs and outputs: in between was the 'black box' – the person. So it is with computers.

Computer people sometimes talk of the GIGO principle: Garbage In = Garbage Out. In practical terms, for you and me, this means that the output from a computer is only as good as the inputs. Inputs occur through the keyboard and output appears on the screen or is printed. All most of us need to know is that we use the keyboard to make inputs and we can read what we write at the keyboard on the screen. We can print out what we have written with a printer and we can store our work on one of a variety of media: floppy disks, hard disks, CD-ROMs, DVDs, etc. There are also other forms of data storage available including small, 'key-ring' attachments that plug into computers for extra storage and portability.

What sort of computer?

Computers come in various shapes and sizes. Although IBM set the standard for today's basic personal computer, various 'clones' have been produced by a wide range of companies. It is possible to shop around and to find real bargains in the computer world. One way to do this is to buy one or more of the various monthly computer magazines, if you can pluck up the courage to wade through the sea of middle-aged men and teenage boys in your local newsagent's. The next sections describe the basic configurations.

It is pointless writing about the finer details of computer chips and sizes. The computer production world is in a constant state of flux. Larger capacity, more compact and cheaper machines seem to be marketed almost every month. What is 'standard' at the time of writing this book is almost certain to be out of date by the time the book is published. Only basic guidelines will be attempted here. As I have suggested above, this is a book about writing and not about computers. The magazines will teach you what you need to know about the innards and keep you up to date.

Theory into practice

Increasingly, patient records are kept on computer and accessed in the wards. Learning to use a computer properly will save you considerable time in the future and make you more efficient in your work.

The basic model

Once, almost all personal computers were of the desktop variety. As the name suggests, these are the sort that sit on your desk. Tower cases have been developed which sit on the floor. Some people are still frightened by computers and worry about breaking them. There is, it turns out, little to break with a computer. You are unlikely to do any lasting damage unless you use a sledgehammer.

The components of a basic desktop computer are:

- **The computer itself**: usually an oblong block containing the central processing unit (CPU), the hard disk and the floppy disk drives and various other bits and pieces that drive the whole unit.
- **The keyboard**: nearly always laid out in the traditional, typewriter mode (with a **QWERTY** keyboard layout). These are now available in various shapes and sizes and some are designed to sit at odd angles to help in the prevention of repetitive strain injury.
- **The mouse**: this is an instrument, with two or three buttons, either attached by wire to the computer or now often wireless. It allows you to press various on-screen buttons that set off certain functions of the application. Most notebook computers have a small pad that emulates a mouse, with two buttons that emulate the mouse buttons. Some notebook computers have a built-in, upside down mouse, known as a tracker ball, whereas other notebooks use a small joystick in the middle of the keyboard for the same set of functions.
- **The visual display unit – the screen**: these come in a range of different degrees of picture resolution and sizes.

This is the traditional computer layout and what most people probably think of when they think of a computer. The advantages of this sort of layout are:

- The keyboard is full-size and allows you to work comfortably.
- The screen is a full-size one and lets you see your work as you write, without too much eyestrain. Larger screens can be purchased which makes the display easier to see.
- The hard disk capacity of such machines is often potentially bigger than is the case with portable computers.

If you are going to buy a computer, want a bargain and have the room, buy a desktop computer – or, if you can afford it, buy a really well-specified laptop PC and use it as your all-round machine.

○━┱ Keywords

QWERTY
The first six letters in a standard keyboard's top row

The laptop

Also known as a notebook in computer terms. The notebook computer is small and light. It is usually about the size of an A4 pad of paper and contains a keyboard, screen, and hard and floppy disk drives. These are usually more expensive than standard PCs but obviously are easily portable. You can fit one inside a briefcase, although they are usually supplied with their own custom-made case. They are the real solution to computing on the move and it is quite possible to carry with you a half-written research report, the whole manuscript of a book, yards of notes and all of your bibliographical references. If you can afford one, think about buying one of these as a second computer. If you really like them, think about one as your *only* computer. These days, the keyboards and screens are improving all the time.

The PDA \ Handheld PC

PDAs (personal digital assistant) and handheld PCs are similar. They are small hand held computers that allow you to perform various functions depending on the model. They are cut down versions of the basic computer model. You can store names and addresses, keep 'to do' lists, have calendar functionality, send and receive email, play music files, use the Internet and word-processing features. They are not really ideal for someone who is going to use a computer primarily for writing purposes.

The tablet PC

The tablet PC has evolved from the laptop. It runs a cut down version of the operating system that a standard computer or laptop would use. (Operating systems are described later in the chapter.) The tablet PC provides most of the performance and functionality of a standard computer. It also provides advanced handwriting and speech recognition capabilities, and a natural interface for entering data using a digital pen in addition to using a keyboard. The tablet PC tends to be very slimline and compact.

Insurance and backups

Portable computers can be stolen. Their portability means that other people can easily remove them and it is quite possible to leave them at stations or airports if you are not used to travelling with them. If you *do* find yourself travelling with a computer (and it can make sense if you take writing seriously but also have to travel), then you need to consider insurance for it. Classe (1995) offers the following pointers for consideration when looking for insurance for portable computers:

- Does your present insurance cover you for habitual use of notebook computers outside the office?
- Are you covered if you take the computer overseas?
- Watch out for exclusion clauses in insurance policies. You may not be covered if you leave a portable in an unattended car – even if it is in the boot. Cover in hotel rooms may depend on the security classification of the hotel. You may not be covered in someone else's office or if you lend your computer to anyone.
- Check excesses on claims. An excess of £250 could end up costing you as much as any repair.

Perhaps most important of all, however, you *must* make backups of all of the data files on a portable. While this rule applies to all computers and computing, it applies even more to portable ones. If your portable computer is stolen, it is unlikely that you will get your essays, dissertation or articles back. If you have access to your computer and you know that you have work on it that is not backed up, get up and back it up now! It is as serious as that. We will look into the subject of backing up your data in more detail later on.

Printers

There are currently three main sorts of printer:

- Inkjet
- Laser
- All in one multifunctional.

Ink jet printer's work by spraying fine bursts of ink on to the page. Sometimes these are bubbles of ink and these printers are then called bubble jet printers. Both are almost silent, fairly speedy, and cheaper to operate than laser printers and cheaper to buy. They have been called the poor person's laser printer. Their only really drawback is that one replaceable cartridge of ink does not print very many pages. This can mean that you pay out quite a lot for new ones and that you may have to break longer printing sessions into small parts. Some companies sell equipment that allows you to replace the ink in the cartridges. These can cut down the cost of using these printers considerably. At the time of writing, ink jet printers offer the best all-round value for money.

Ink jet printers are available in a colour option at only a relatively small increase in price. Most writers probably will not need a colour printer but, increasingly, colour work is being used in the production of charts and diagrams and may soon be an integral part of most postgraduate dissertations and theses.

The laser printer is the one to go for if you can afford it. They work in a similar way to photocopiers and are very quick, easy to use and almost silent in operation. They produce a very high quality printout and the end product looks very professional.

The all in one multifunctional combines printer, copier, scanner and fax machine, all in one 'box'. Some of these are remarkably cheap, for the technology involved, and work very well. If you have a requirement for the extra functionality these machines are well worth considering.

Buying a computer for writing

What computer should you buy? Computer hardware (the keyboard, monitor and computing unit itself) is changing rapidly. It is also dropping in price. Any specific advice about particular models of computer would be out of place. Certain general suggestions may be made. A computer for use in the home that is not going to age too quickly should fulfil most and perhaps all of the following criteria:

● It should have a monitor and keyboard that suit you. On the monitor issue, a larger screen is ideal for word-processing. A large-size screen allows you to see and work on a whole A4 page of print at a time. Obviously, larger screens also cost more and are 'non-standard'. There are currently many LCD (liquid crystal display) screens available. These are thinner, flat screens that take up a lot less desk space than the more conventional bigger, bulkier ones. They are also more ecologically friendly. Similarly, the 'feel' of a keyboard is the subject of much debate. Some prefer a keyboard that reminds them of a typewriter and 'clicks' when the keys are pressed. Others prefer a 'deader' keyboard. There are also ergonomically friendly keyboards that are produced to specifically reduce the risk of repetitive strain injury. These are angled in a specific way to make your wrists feel more comfortable. It is recommended that you try typing on a range of keyboards before you choose yours. This is one of the problems when buying computers through the post. Unless you have had experience of the model that you order, you will not be able to try out the keyboard before you buy. I suspect, though, that the keyboard question is only an issue when you first buy a computer. After a couple of weeks, you get used to the feel of the keyboard and no longer worry about whether or not it 'clicks'. I work on a range of keyboards in my job and I don't find any of them particularly objectionable – and I touch-type.

- It should come with a backup device. Many computers are now sold with some form of backup device as part of the package. A CD writer for example, which operates as a CD Rom drive but also allows you to copy data to CDs which you can store away from the computer. Other options include a zip drive or a USB drive which plugs into the computer and again allows data to be transferred. New backup devices are being produced all the time but as long as you are aware of the importance of such a device you can ask for advice at the time of purchase.

- It should come with a device to connect it to the Internet. This is important as you will be able to gain huge benefits from being connected to the Internet. You can research almost any subject, contact people via email and submit work electronically. Almost every computer that is sold today will come with such a device but take advice on the options for your particular circumstance. For example, if you intend to use the Internet a lot and there is a digital exchange in your area you can purchase an option to have a much faster Internet connection.

- It should come with a decent warranty and support options. If something does go wrong with the computer you will want it fixed as soon as possible with the minimum of stress. Most manufacturers and suppliers will provide some sort of warranty. The best ones to go for are those with 2 or 3 years on site maintenance that will cover parts and labour for any defects in the computer hardware. A free telephone support help line is also useful to troubleshoot minor problems. Beware of those telephone lines that charge a certain amount per minute.

Where do I buy it?

There are a number of ways of buying a computer. First, though, you need to choose which one you are going to buy. If you already have one and are upgrading, you are likely to know what sort you want. In the end, there is little to choose between the various makes in terms of quality. These days, nearly all computers are of high quality. You will pay extra for the big names as they tend to use higher quality components. You will also pay extra for on-site, good maintenance. You may also pay extra for telephone help. In my experience, the latter is vital. For some reason, I have never yet been able to make a printer work with a computer, first time.

Talk to people who know about computers before you buy one. While they often have odd favourites and can be a rather quirky crowd, they can usually offer good advice about what to buy. If you know what you want, it is safe and usually much cheaper to buy via the Internet or mail order. These days, you can ring up with a credit card and the machinery is installed in your home by the end of the week. It will be fully set up and configured by the company and usually you will be able to secure on-site maintenance if anything goes wrong.

If you are not sure what you want, many companies will offer a pre-sales service, which will give free advice. All the large manufacturers have their own web sites and you can obtain quotes for the computer either online or by calling pre sales. Get a few quotes to compare what is being offered – usually it is the after sales package which will differ as you will find the hardware can be tailored to your individual circumstances. You can also go to a dedicated computer shop or manufacturer outlet. These are often away from the high street but sell nothing except computers and computer-related goods. They can offer the same service as the mail order firms and are usually only a little more expensive.

Key points **Top tips**

- Consider buying a laptop, rather than a desktop computer. This will mean you can work wherever you want to
- Consider buying from one of the more well known PC manufacturers. They usually provide better after sales support options
- Learn to type.

The Internet

The Internet, cyberspace, and the information superhighway: these are all terms that students, managers and clinicians have grown used to. They refer to a huge 'network of networks' – a worldwide linking up of computers and computer networks.

The Internet has changed the way many people handle and process information. Just a brief look at the things you can do with the Internet can give a clue to how managers, educators and students can use the system. First, they have access to huge amounts of information – from papers, books and files. Second, they are able to make contact with lots of like-minded people who share their research, management or clinical interests. They can search for publications, contact specialists in other countries and even set up international 'real time' conferences.

So what do you need to access the Internet? A computer, a device to connect to the Internet and a service provider. After that, it is a question of learning how to negotiate your way around the Internet. This is where some reading matter can help.

E-mail and writing

Students are able to type their essays and projects on the computer, save the file and then e-mail it to their teachers for marking. Also, e-mail is an ideal way of students keeping in touch with their fellow students and with staff members. Some colleges offer a form of counselling via e-mail. Most students will find it beneficial to open an e-mail account. Most service providers that provide Internet access also provide email accounts. Many of these allow you to access your e-mail from any computer attached to the net. This is a point worth checking when you choose an email provider.

Also, you have to be a little bit careful about the *way* in which you write e-mails. Perhaps because they are written very quickly and because they may include abbreviations, they are subject to being misunderstood. It is remarkably easy to offend people with a not-very-well written e-mail. There is a certain email etiquette, which you will become more familiar with as you use it. For example the most common mistake people make is writing in block capitals. This is regarded as a very angry form of text within e-mail and is used to stress a point vigorously.

Increasingly, of course, people are also communicating, in writing, through texting on mobile phones. Extreme brevity is often used in texts ('u', instead of 'you', for example). However, you should be careful not to carry these abbreviations into your college or research work. Again, it remains to be seen whether or not these abbreviations will, over time, be incorporated into 'formal' writing.

Software

Your computer, on its own, will be of no use to you. You will need to have applications to run on it. These are discussed in this section of the chapter. Make sure, though, that you have an 'operating system' already on your hard disk when you buy your machine. Almost all new computers will come with this pre installed. An operating system is the basic software that provides an interface for you to interact with your computer. The most frequently used operating system is Microsoft® Windows (although Linux is an alternative). There are many different versions of Microsoft Windows. An updated version tends to be produced every few years. Each version is fairly similar to use but with new functionality being added. Ask for the latest version of Windows to be installed when you purchase your computer.

Once an operating system has been installed on your machine, you can forget about it. It fires up when you switch on and it works away in the background without your having to think very much about it. If you want to, and if you like that sort of thing, you can also spend a lifetime learning all about the ins and outs of your operating system. It is probably better to spend the time *writing* on the computer.

Word-processing applications

The most important computer application for the writer is the word processor. Word-processing applications for the personal computer come in many shapes and sizes. As a minimum, you want one that can perform the following functions:

- Count words
- Number pages
- Spell check
- Move text around
- Set margins
- Show text on the screen in roughly the same format as you will see it on the printed page. If you use modern word-processing

applications, you will see the text almost exactly as it appears on paper. This is called WYSIWYG – What you See Is What You Get.

Also, you want a word processor that is easy to use. Most take a little time to learn and some of the larger ones have huge numbers of functions. In my experience, people tend to think that they will not want all the extra functions. For everyday use, this is true. There comes a time, though, when you *will* use some of the more esoteric functions. Examples of these other functions include:

- The ability to sort lines or paragraphs of text, alphabetically or by number
- The ability to use bullets such as the ones in this list
- The ability to work with more than one document at once
- The ability to create indexes
- The ability to work with very long textual documents
- The ability to change font sizes
- The ability to create 'macros', keyboard shortcuts that allow you to access some of the more complicated aspects of the word-processing application
- The use of a thesaurus for checking and changing words
- The use of a **bolding** facility that prints blacker characters
- The ability to import graphical images
- The ability to import spreadsheet tables
- The ability to apply pre-set 'styles' to a document to make sure that it is laid out consistently.

The list can go on. Only the larger commercial word-processing applications are likely to contain all these functions. For me, the important things in considering what word processor to buy are these:

- Ease of use
- Range of functions.

What follows is a brief review of some of the better known word-processing packages. The important thing is to find the package that you are most comfortable with. Most word-processor users tend to think that the one that they use is the best. I admit to being a Microsoft® Word® fan and I am constantly surprised at what it can do. Four years on, I am still learning some of its more rarely used functions but when I do need them, I usually find that they are easy to use. There seems to be a critical period in learning to use a word-processing application. Somehow, you need to spend time getting the hang of the 'whole' of the application. Once you have this overall feel for how the application operates, you seem to relax and are able to take a more leisurely approach to some of the finer details.

The particular virtue of Windows applications is that they all look fairly similar on the screen. This means that switching from one application to another is much easier than it used to be. If you can learn one Windows application, you can easily learn others. Also, it is easy to transfer files across from one word-processing application to another. Most of the main Windows word processors have the facility for saving a file in the format of another. This is particularly useful if you are working on a project with another person who is using a different application.

Microsoft® Word®

Microsoft Word is a fully featured word-processing package and one that is ideal for writers. There are many different versions of Word, updated versions appear periodically. The latest versions tend to be backward compatible, which means that they will open files created in earlier versions of Word. Apart from all the usual word-processing features that we will explore in the next chapter, Word allows you to work with multiple documents. You might, for example, want to work with a variety of versions of an essay or an article and the application allows you to switch, quickly, between the various versions. The application also has a very versatile 'undo' feature. As you work at polishing your essay or report, you may find that you don't like the last series of 'edits' that you made. Using the undo feature, you can quickly 'take off' the editing (and, just as easily, 'put back' the editing).

The application is very easy to customise, according to how you work. You can set up the usual range of 'macros' (or short cuts). You can also develop 'toolbars' – sets of buttons that sit at the top of the screen that allow you to perform certain functions quickly. For example, on the toolbar I am using to write these words, I have buttons to do the following:

- Set up the subheading styles
- Count the words in a whole document
- Select all the text in a document (this is one way to make 'global' changes to a document)
- Find and replace selections of text
- Call up a copy of my CV
- Insert the full name and 'path' of a document as a footnote on every page

- Call up the file that contains the manuscript of this book (when the book is finished and the publishers are happy with the manuscript, this button will be taken off the toolbar).

With many versions of Word you can also illustrate and generally 'dress up' your work. You can do the following:

- Generate graphs, histograms and pie charts
- Use 'clip art' to illustrate news letters and projects
- Generate charts for use as overhead projections in teaching
- Draw organisation charts.

A good word-processing application can help to make your work look more professional and can help you to communicate your thoughts through iconic representation. A basic rule applies here, though: keep it simple. Generally, communication is much clearer if you stick to simple charts and representations.

WordPerfect®

WordPerfect is another fully featured word processor and contains many of the features that can be found in Word. It does, however, have quite a different 'feel' to Word and many of the functions work in different ways. Like most Windows word processors, however, it has the familiar pull-down menus at the top of the screen and rows of buttons that can be customised. It also has an excellent file-handling system that allows you to preview files before you open them. This is particularly useful if you are not sure of the name that you gave to a file and want to have a quick look at the file in question before you open it up on the screen.

There are lots of other word-processing packages that you may want to explore.

Other applications for the writer

This is not intended to be an exhaustive list, just to demonstrate some of the range of electronic tools available to the writer.

The suite of applications

There are a number of packages on the market that supply you with a whole range of applications bundled together. These are known as suites and usually contain a fully featured word processor, a spreadsheet, a database and a graphics application. At the moment, the most well known packages are Microsoft® Office® and Lotus SmartSuite®. This is an ideal way to buy a number of important applications together. Buying a suite is always cheaper than buying the individual applications separately and the companies that make these suites will often offer special prices to induce people to change from one company's applications to another. If you are a WordPerfect user, for example, you will probably be able to 'cross platforms' to Microsoft Office for a remarkably cheap price.

The point, obviously, is that you need to know that you are going to *use* the other applications before you buy a suite. Spreadsheets are ideal if you are going to be working with numbers – a spreadsheet is a huge matrix of 'rows and columns' and it allows you to manipulate figures in all sorts of ways. Databases are likely to be useful to most writers and can be used to store all sorts of structured information, from bibliographical references to names and addresses. Graphics applications are also useful to the technical writer. While most word-processing applications allow you to produce bar charts, histograms and graphs, dedicated graphics applications usually allow you to do these things better. If you want to illustrate your work in other ways, too, you will make use of a graphics package.

The alternative to the suite is the integrated package. Integrated packages are applications that contain features of word processors, spreadsheets, databases and graphics applications all in the one application. Whereas a suite is a set of discrete applications (which can usually work together), the integrated package is one application containing 'cut down' aspects of the larger applications. Examples of integrated packages include Microsoft® Works®.

Edmunds (1995) offers the following buyer's checklist for the person who is considering buying a suite of applications or an integrated package:

- If you are considering buying more than one mainstream application from the same publisher, you should probably consider buying the suite
- Integrated packages require less computer resources than software suites but include fewer features – check that any features you require are included
- If you expect to make a lot of use of one particular application in the integrated package, say a word-processing application, you will be better off buying the full version rather than relying on a reduced feature set
- Special suite prices are available from all vendors when upgrading from a competitive or earlier product
- At under £100, integrated packages are exceptional value, but skimping on software if you really need the feature sets of complete applications may not pay off in the long term.

Anti Virus Software \ Firewall

Viruses are malicious programs that can cause damage to your computer operating system and personal data. There are many different types of virus and they spread in many different ways. The most important thing from your point of view is that you are protected from viruses with adequate anti virus software. Anti virus software once installed will remain active, constantly searching for viruses. Software updates are available via the Internet so that as new viruses are produced, you can update your virus-checker accordingly. These tend to be produced weekly or as soon as a high risk virus appears. Two of the most popular anti virus software applications are Mcafee and Norton. Most new computers will come with anti virus software pre-installed but you will need to check that this is the case.

A firewall is a program that sits in between your computer and the Internet and filters out harmful attacks on your machine. It can trap viruses and stop others accessing your computer from the Internet. The latest operating systems have built-in firewalls. Firewalls are also commonly shipped as part of an anti virus solution. Once again it is worth checking what you are buying.

Spreadsheets

A spreadsheet application allows you to develop a huge 'rows and columns' chart on your computer. It does more than this: it also allows you to undertake a whole range of calculations on each or on a selection of the rows and columns. In some ways it is like a computerised and automated accounts book. On the other hand, it can also do far more than just compute rows and columns. It can be used for at least the following functions too:

- For storing addresses
- For compiling bibliographies and reference lists
- For drawing 'word illustrations' in column format
- For computing frequency counts
- For working out means and modes.

Figure 3.1 (overleaf) is an example of what a spreadsheet looks like when it has data in it:

Examples of spreadsheet applications that are currently available commercially include:

- Microsoft® Excel®
- Lotus 123

	A	B	C	D
1	Response to Question 6 (Health care professionals should receive more training in the field of child abuse).			
2		Social workers	Doctors	Nurses
3	Agree	23	37	56
4	Disagree	10	8	10
5	Don't know	0	3	5

Figure 3.1 *Example of part of a spreadsheet*

Other application software

This section looks at individual software packages that are widely used and may well be of interest to the writer.

Endnote Plus

Endnote Plus is an application designed for working with bibliographical references. What does it do? Talking through a typical application of the program is probably the best way of describing how EndNote Plus works in practice.

Here is one way of using it. Imagine that you are working on an essay or a paper in your word-processing application. You want to support an argument with a reference but you cannot quite remember the particular article or book. You call up EndNote Plus and browse through your reference collection. Finding the right paper, you mark it, press a couple of buttons to transfer the reference to the application's 'clipboard' and then you return to your word-processing application. You then press another couple of buttons and a note about the reference is pasted straight into your essay.

When you have finished working through your essay or paper in this way – collecting references from EndNote Plus as you work – you then have to think about how the reference list at the end of your paper will be formatted. You may, for example, want to use the Vancouver referencing system. On the other hand, the journal to which you are submitting your paper may lay down very specific instructions about how to list your references. All of this presents no problem to EndNote Plus. At the end of your paper you simply ask the application to format your reference list in any one of a wide range of referencing styles, including all the main 'academic' ones and many of the most common journal styles.

Now imagine another possibility. You send your paper off to the journal but it is not accepted for publication. You modify it a little and then submit it to another. Before you do that, you realise that the new journal requires another style of referencing. Again, this presents no problems. EndNote Plus allows you simply to change all the references and your final list to suit the requirements of the second journal. In theory you could go on doing this *ad nauseam*.

EndNote Plus offers an incredible amount of flexibility in storing, sorting, searching and organising your reference collection. It will also generate files for transferring information to other applications and will work 'automatically' with Microsoft Word and WordPerfect. It is also fully compatible with EndNote and EndNote Plus on the Apple Macintosh.

Reference collections are both personal and valuable. This application not only helps you to cite references in papers and articles, it also encourages you to build your own reference library. Not only of books and papers but also of computer software and other forms of 'text'. You can do simple and complex searches and build reference collections up to 32,000 entries long. It would make an ideal institutional as well as a personal purchase. It comes with a very well written manual and a large number of preset 'forms' for entering your references. If you do not like the ones you find, you can make your own. It is worth spending some time learning to use this application to its limit. It will be time well spent and will quickly be repaid by the time and energy you save when you start using the application as a writing aid.

Microsoft® Project®

Developing and planning long- and short-term projects used to involve graph paper and complicated wall charts. Now you can get your projects organised, much more efficiently, with a computer application. Microsoft Project is what it says: an application for organising all elements of any type of project. Health-care professionals are likely to find it particularly useful for organising research projects, organisational change, long-term management development, trials, conferences and curriculum plans.

There are three phases to project management. First, you create the project. This is, traditionally, the 'brainstorming' phase. Project allows you to play around with possibilities and then to structure a framework for organising the project. Second, you manage the project. Project allows you to keep track of all the elements of your project, to predict problems, to reallocate time and make all sorts of fine adjustments. Third, you produce reports of the project. Again, Project helps here by creating informative and attractive reports quickly and easily.

The project management techniques that Project offers are comprehensive. You can use the critical path method of scheduling – an approach already in use by many managers. Or you can use the application evaluation review technique (PERT) – another method that has often been used in the health-care professions to organise and manage the use of time. Finally, you can use Gantt charts – perhaps the most familiar way of illustrating time-spans in a project.

Initially, you can enter 'events' in your project into a spreadsheet-type screen. Then you can reorder events, retime them, reschedule them and manipulate those events to a considerable degree. Various views of your data allow you different perspectives on your project. The business of working with Project takes you far beyond a mere paper exercise. The application can help you develop and think-through both large and small projects. Fund-holders will appreciate being able to time and cost sections of projects and know that they can always run projects of the 'what-if?' sort.

This is not an application to load up and work with immediately. You have to invest a little effort in getting to know it. Fortunately, as with many Microsoft® applications, a good deal of help is at hand. First, you get a run-through of the main points of the application when you first start it up. Then, you can have the application 'talk you though' the various elements of project design and scheduling. Finally, you can call up context-sensitive help at any time. Also, the documentation is excellent and informative. Microsoft produces readable help material that is not simply alphabetical lists of what applications do. Instead, it is laid out in easy-to-follow and easy-to-digest sections.

Project is highly compatible with other Windows applications and particularly with other Microsoft applications. If you already use Microsoft Word or Microsoft Excel, you will soon get used to Project. It employs the common user interface that runs throughout the Microsoft range of applications and honours all the 'Windows conventions'.

Microsoft® Publisher®

Publisher is an application which lets you create many different documents and publications. You can create leaflets, posters, newsletters, postcards and artwork etc. You can also merge pictures and text, which can be useful for the writer.

Microsoft® PowerPoint®

PowerPoint is an application that allows you to create presentations. It allows you to create slides and add text, graphics, animation and multimedia video clips. You can also use it to create slide shows.

File retrieval software

Everyone does it at some point. You press a couple of wrong keys and suddenly the file you are working on disappears for ever. You stab wildly at the keyboard. You repeat a series of keystrokes over and over again like a rat in a psychologist's laboratory. Nothing brings your file back. At this point, you may decide that computers are not for you.

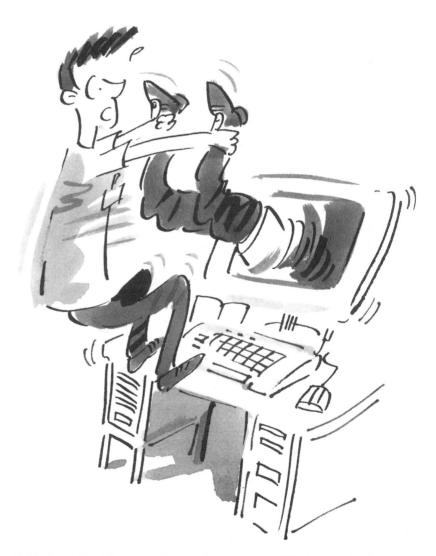

Retrieving deleted files is much easier if you have specially developed software.

Or you may burst into tears. You could reach for file retrieval software. This software can rescue deleted files and even deleted disks. As someone who once deleted a complete book chapter I was working on, I only wish that I had this software 3 years ago.

A writer's software starter kit

So what *must* you have in the way of software? This chapter has offered descriptions of quite a few applications: it is sometimes difficult to know what sorts of application are absolutely essential. Here is a shortlist of applications recommended for anyone who wants to set their computer up for writing.

A word-processing application

Clearly essential. You are not going to write very much with your computer if you do not have one of these. As we have seen, there is a considerable range to choose from. If you are new to computing, one of the 'smaller' ones will be quite adequate and you may even find that the application Write – which is supplied with Windows – is sufficient. It can certainly enable you to carry out all the basic functions of producing, editing and printing out documents.

A simple database application

You will want to store bibliographical references as you write. As we have seen, you can use a variety of applications for this purpose. Simplicity is probably the keyword here. What you do not want to do is to have to learn a complicated application simply in order to file away your references. Various applications have been described in this chapter and a number of dedicated bibliographical applications are available as shareware (see page 57).

An anti-virus application and a firewall

These are essential if you use the Internet from your computer on a regular basis. They will prevent viruses from attacking your machine and keep 'intruders' out.

Copyright

Remember that all software is copyright. You cannot simply borrow someone else's disks and then copy them on to your machine. If you are going to use an application you must buy it. Mostly, the copyright agreement on software is rather like the copyright attached to books. Only one person at a time can read a book and you must not photocopy it. The same goes for software. Only one person at a time should be able to use a particular application.

Shareware

Shareware has a unique marketing strategy. A shareware application is distributed free of charge (although a charge is usually made for the disks and the handling). The idea is that you first try the application and then, if you like it, you send away a registration fee to use the application. In the first instance, you usually have between 30 and 90 days to try out the application before you register it. Further, during this time, you are encouraged to make copies of the application for your colleagues and friends. Then, the same principles apply: they are allowed to try out the application and then send off to become registered users if they find it useful.

The advantages of the shareware approach are many for the home PC user. First, the user gets a chance to try the application before making a financial commitment to it. Second, the registration fees for shareware are considerably cheaper than buying copies of most commercial applications. Also, the quality of shareware applications is improving all the time and some of the best are easily the equal of commercial software. Finally, shareware offers you the easy approach to learning more about computer applications and exploring a variety of methods of working with data that might not be available to you if you had to rely on buying commercial packages. The names and addresses of shareware distributors are available in any of the monthly computer magazines. Such magazines often include one or two shareware applications on a 'free' disk attached to the front cover.

Shareware is not free. The idea, as noted above, is to try out the application, decide if you like it and then pay for it. If you decide not to use the application then you can simply give the disks to another person or format the disks for use with other files. The only free applications are those available in the public domain. These public domain applications are often distributed by the same people who handle shareware, although it is often not made clear in their catalogues what is shareware and what is in the public domain.

RRRRRRapid recap

Check your progress so far by working through the following questions.

1. What are the four main types of computer?
2. What software is recommended for writers?
3. Why is it important to install a firewall on to your computer?

If you have difficulty with more than one of the questions, read through the section again to refresh your understanding before moving on.

References

Classe, A. (1995) Portable peace of mind. *PC Direct*, January.

Edmunds, N. (1995) Suite success. *PC Direct*, January.

4

Writing with a computer

There is no such thing as a moral or an immoral book. Books are well written, or badly written.

Oscar Wilde

The point is to write. Computers may seem to take away some of the romance and the mystery of writing but they can help you no end. The previous chapter offered reasons for using a computer in writing and described some of the software that is available for personal computers. In this chapter, we identify some of the issues related to writing with the use of a computer. It is assumed that you have chosen your word-processing program and that you have got used to the fundamentals of it. You have, perhaps, passed the stage that the writer Primo Levi describes as he writes of beginning to use a computer and word processor:

> If I now analyse my initial anxiety, I realise that it was in great part illogical: it contained an old fear of those who write, the fear that the unique, inestimable text worked at so hard, which will give you eternal fame, might be stolen or end up in a manhole. Here you write, the words appear neatly on the screen, well aligned, but they are shadows: they are immaterial, deprived of the reassuring support of the paper. The written word speaks out: the screen does not; when you are satisfied with the text 'you put it on disk', where it becomes invisible. Is it still there, absconding in some little corner of the memory disk, or did you destroy it with some mistaken move?

Levi 1989

Housekeeping

The word, in this context, is used to denote those activities that are concerned with the management of computer files and the hard disk. Think of the computer as being a digital filing cabinet.

When you start using the software we have discussed in the last chapter, for example the word processor – you will begin creating files. Files are the name given to the work that you create and save onto the computer. If you write a letter and then save it onto your hard disk drive you will be prompted to give it a name – so that you can easily find and identify it for future reference. This is a file name and the letter is known as a word processing file. It is tempting, when you first get a computer with a hard disk, to simply pile all your software on to it in no particular order. This is fatal. If you do this, it will be difficult to find specific files. Instead, you should make use of the hierarchical faculty of the operating system that you are using.

Files can be stored on the computer in places called 'folders'. These are created and named by you. This helps to classify the files even further. For example if you have created files that are letters, you may wish to create a folder called `Letters` to store them in. If you have also written a number of reports you can create a folder called `Reports` to store the report files in.

It makes sense to store all your folders in the same place so that each time you wish to open, edit or save a file it will be easy to find. Most versions of the Microsoft Windows operating system have a main file already created called `My Documents`. It is generally stored on the desktop of the operating system, so when you switch the computer on and it finishes starting up you will be able to see the My Documents folder. It is good practice to use this as your root folder and create sub folders of your own classification within it. Then store your files within these folders and they will all be in one place.

Going back to the analogy of the computer as being a digital filing cabinet – the My Documents folder would be the cabinet itself, the sub folders you create within it would be the folders within the cabinet and the files you create would be the files that sit in the folders of the cabinet. Once you start creating files and saving them, this process will become a lot easier to understand but it is important that you have an understanding about creating and storing files and folders from the outset. If you are uncertain about how to do this, consult the help documentation that accompanies your operating system or your programs.

Figure 4.1 illustrates this set of relationships.

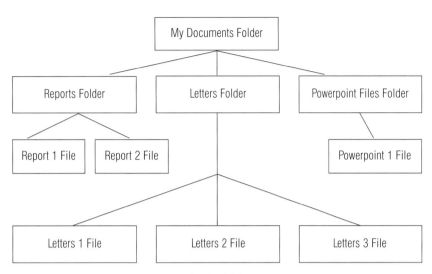

Figure 4.1 *One possible hierarchy for the folders on a computer*

Housekeeping also covers making sure that you know what is on your hard disk. Make frequent checks to see what files you have made and which ones you *have* to keep on your hard disk. Do not keep files on the hard disk that you never use.

Theory into practice

If you use a shared computer (in the ward, or the university department), do not change any of the settings. It is important that *everyone* who uses the computer knows what to expect from it.

Most of all, housekeeping refers to the process of backing up your data. Put simply, this means that everything that is within your personal folders (the filing cabinet that you have created) should also be on other media. All your program files will already be on portable media for that is the medium on which you bought them. It is a good idea to get into the habit of backing up at the end of each working session on the computer. Programs are available that will back up any new files that have been made, automatically. All you have to do is to invoke the program, put a new disk in the appropriate drive and press a couple of buttons. The program will then do what is called an 'incremental' backup. The only files that are backed up are new ones or ones that have been written to since the last backup. Alternatively, many programs have backup facilities. WordPerfect, for example, allows you to back-up files through its 'file manager' feature. All you have to do is to highlight any new or modified files and ask for copies to be made to floppy disk.

If you purchased a specific backup device as recommended, one of the first things to do when you have set up your computer is to learn how to use it. Backup devices come in different forms, for example zip disks, CD writers or USB hard disk drives. When your data has been transferred you are safe in the knowledge that if something goes wrong with your computer, or if it is stolen, then your work is not lost.

Backing up your personal data is essential and the importance of this cannot be stressed enough. Many hard disks fail at some time, and if one does, you stand to lose all the files that are on it. If you back up your work, you can always find the files and the work that you need. That work is always ready elsewhere, even when you cannot use the hard disk.

Setting up your word processor

Most of the larger word processors can be configured to work the way you want them to. They all have 'default' settings: standard settings that allow you to work with the program straight away. On the other hand, you can change many of these defaults in order to have the word processor work the way *you* want it. Examples of defaults that you can reset and have running with new definitions include the following:

- **Colours**. The rule, as ever, is simplicity. Do not overwhelm yourself with too many colour combinations. Use the same colour to indicate various degrees of 'large' fonts. Don't allocate a different colour to each function or you will quickly forget what your colour scheme means. Also, have a change of background colour occasionally.

- **Right and left margins**. You can have wide settings for these when you are working at the screen and then change them for printing out. The wide margins when you are working will allow your eyes to scan a single line at a time and thus save you constantly turning your head back and forward. Also, some word-processing programs cause the writing to go off the edge of the screen if you use only 2 cm margins. Reset them so that you can see all of what you have written.

- **Top and bottom margins**. For work that you submit for publication, allow fairly generous margins all round. I have mine set to 3 cm for top, bottom and sides.

- **Tab settings**. The correct setting for 'indents' at the beginning of paragraphs is 1 or 1.5 'ems'. An em is the width of a single letter m. It is possible on some word processors to set the first tab setting to ensure that all your indents are 1 or 1.5 ems.

- **Back-up settings**. Modern word processors automatically back up the file that you are working on to the hard disk, at pre-set intervals. You can set the time limit for this. You must *still* make regular backups of your personal data.

- **Font sizes**. Most word processors allow you to work in different-sized letters and numbers. With some, you may see the difference on the screen.

- **Underlining style: words and spaces or just words**. It is usual to underline both words and spaces. If you are printing out on a laser printer, you may prefer to use italics rather than underlining in your work. In a manuscript, underlining is used to represent passages that will be printed as italics in the final publication. I have changed my 'underlining' command on my word processor to produce italics automatically. This stops me having to think whether or not I want underlining or italics. Nothing is for ever: the underlining function can soon be returned to normal if this should be important at a later date.

- **Paper and page size**. There is only one size of paper for writing: A4. Do not use smaller or larger sizes. Also, buy fairly good paper of about 80 gsm in weight. For posting work to publishers, do not use heavier paper than this otherwise your bill for stamps will be rather large. Use plain paper and not 'laid'. Laid paper has faint lines running through it in the style of a watermark.

- **Page numbering.**

- **Headers and footers and the contents of these**. Use these sparingly. Although printed books and magazines have running headers and footers it is not a good idea to use them in manuscripts that you send to editors. They only have to cross them through when they are editing your work. On the other hand, with book manuscripts, it is good practice to have a simple header that contains your name and the title of the book. This is useful if the editor or anyone else leaves half of your manuscript in the office and half at home. Without any sort of identification, it may be difficult to marry the two piles of paper together.

- **Keyboard layout**. Some word processors allow you to modify your keyboard considerably.

- **Justification**. You may prefer to have both margins flush or to have the words at the right margin 'ragged'.

- **Column and/or table settings**.
- **Line spacing**. If you are submitting work for publication, always double-space it.
- Buttons. Many Windows word-processing packages allow you to set up 'buttons' at the top of the screen which, when 'pressed' with the mouse, trigger certain functions. Examples of buttons you could have on your 'button bar' include: 1) a button that opens up the file you are working on; 2) a button that automatically saves your work to the hard disk; 3) a button that saves a copy of your work to a removable disk; 4) a button that counts the words in your file; and many more.

Many word processors allow you to write 'macros'. Consider, for a moment, a function of your word processor that requires you to work through lots of keystrokes in order to invoke the function. A macro is a 'shorthand' that allows you to assign all of those keystrokes to just one or two keystrokes. For example, on the keyboard that I am working on at present, if I press ALT and S, the word processor will run the spell-checker. These key-presses are not standard: first I had to write the macros that make them function in that way. It is possible to build up a considerable collection of such macros that allow you to invoke functions quickly and easily. It is worth taking a little time to learn the macro language that accompanies your word processor.

With some word processors it is also possible to reassign keys to function according to your own preference. None of this is irreversible. Don't get nervous about what could happen if you make mistakes. It is always possible to reinstate the normal function of the keys that you change.

Key points | **Top tips**

Write quickly, straight into the computer: edit slowly
- Back up your work to a disk or other medium
- Send your work by e-mail, if you can, and save paper and time.

Working with a word-processing program

There are a number of tips that can make writing easier with a word-processing program. These are itemised below. Try to standardise the way that you work so that your output is consistent. If you decide, for example, to use 5 cm margins when you write

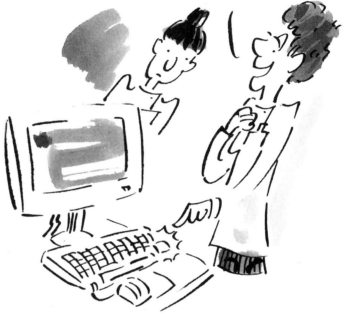

Oh yes, I just press this key and the computer writes my essay, adds the references and switches the kettle on.

Macros are a useful way of shortcutting certain functions, which can save you time.

essays, *always* use 5 cm margins. Consider resetting the margin defaults to 5 cm, so that every piece of writing you produce has 5 cm margins. This sort of standardisation is important. Here are the tips for working with your word-processing program:

- Although your final output will usually be in double-spaced lines, use single-spaced lines to work with on your screen. Double-line spacing on the monitor means that you effectively halve the amount of text you can see on the screen at any one time.
- Work with small documents. You do not need to keep the whole of a piece of work in one file. Large documents including artwork and tables may take time to work through. It may be better to split a large document into two separate files.
- When working on large documents, work in Normal view rather than Page view, as this will allow you scan lines of text more easily.

- Be consistent in your use of underlining, bolding and italics. Don't mix the three. Settle for one type of emphasis and stick to it.
- Be consistent in your line spacing between ends of sections and new subheadings. As a rule, leave two lines between the end of a section and a new subheading. Then leave one line between the subheading and the text. You can also set up heading styles within your document so that this is done automatically.
- Be careful about indenting paragraphs. Do not indent the first paragraph of a piece of work, or subsequent first paragraphs under subheadings. After that, indent every paragraph. For an immediate example of both line spacing and indentation, look at the use of both in this book.
- Be consistent with your use of full stops and commas. It is not always necessary to use punctuation in a 'bullet' list (such as this one). If you do use them, use them consistently.
- Avoid mixing up different fonts on a page. It is not good practice to use all the different sizes of numbers and figures that your word processor will allow. Keep to one or two sizes. As a rule, 12 pt is a good size of font to use for everyday writing. Also, Times Roman is a clear and clean font if you have a laser printer. Fashions in typeface come and go. At the moment, sans serif fonts (those without 'tails' on the letters) tend to be out of fashion for large blocks of text, although they are good for headings as they are clean and simple. **This is an example of a sans serif font.** Times Roman seems to be something of a standard font.
- Don't overuse graphics. If your word processor can use 'clip art' or pre-drawn pieces of drawing and illustration, use it very sparingly, if at all.
- If you work in more than one document at a time and have a coloured screen, change the background colours in the second and third document screens. In this way, you are less likely to be muddled up about which document you are working on.
- Save your work regularly. That means that you have to stop typing and consciously save your work to the hard disk. Again, later on, backup your personal data so that you always have a copy of it. If you do lose a document through a power cut or similar, there is an auto recover feature built into certain operating systems. This means the computer may have saved a temporary version of the

file as you were working on it that can be retrieved if something goes wrong. Consult your operating system guide for more information on this feature.

- Use 'odd' names for temporary files that you use for blocks of text or for ideas. I tend to use the file names 'Dog' and 'Cat' for these sorts of files. When I am 'housekeeping' I know that these are files that I can delete.

- If you are referring to names of authors and dates while writing essays or articles, and cannot remember those names and dates as you write, use a consistent symbol to note the place where they should go. I use three asterisks (***). Then, using the 'search' facility, you can go straight to those symbols after you have finished writing and fill in the blanks. Thus, when I am writing, a section of the text may look like this: 'Student-centred learning owes much to the work of Carl Rogers (***). The idea that adult learners might want to be responsible for their learning was also discussed by Malcolm Knowles (***) and Postman and Weingartner (***).' Then I simply search for the ***s and insert the correct dates.

- Write quickly and edit later. If you find that your spelling suffers a little, don't worry too much; you can always correct this with the spell checker. If this seems a sloppy approach, remember: the word processor is there to save you time – use it. If you find it helps, use shorthand for words that you find difficult to spell. For instance, you might use 'exp' for the term 'experiential', if you find that word tricky to spell. When you have finished writing, the spell checker will soon flag this 'non-word' up and you will be offered the correct spelling for it. It is quite possible to become much faster at writing through developing a personal shorthand of this sort.

- A variant of the above is to use letters for complicated names. For example, if you are writing an essay about Dostoevsky but find the name difficult to spell and remember, simply type the letters DY. Then use the search and replace command to replace those letters with the full name throughout your manuscript.

- It is also a very good idea to put all the ways you often normally misspell words into your word processor's Auto correct (if it has one), so that the program automatically knows which word you intended and corrects it as you go along.

- Try to learn most of the functions of your word processor and learn all the shortcuts. I once found a colleague working through a file on the screen, inserting 'hard returns' between each line of text to ensure that the manuscript printed out in double spacing. He did not realise that he could set the program to print in double spacing.

- If your word processor has a thesaurus, use it regularly to give you ideas for different words. This cannot only teach you words but can freshen your writing.

- Avoid footnotes and endnotes in documents, even if your word processing program can handle them automatically. If you have anything that you want to put as a footnote, incorporate it into the main body of the text. Otherwise, leave it out altogether. Footnotes are always distracting. An exception to this rule is discussed in Chapter 8.

- If you can, run off a draft 'hard' copy (i.e. a printed copy) of your work before you submit it. It is often easier to spot typographical errors on the printed page than it is on the computer screen.

- Don't work for long periods at the computer. If you *have* to, work on different documents. It is a great strain to both eyes and posture if you work for hours on one document. Look away from the screen when the computer is busy working at a particular function. Get used to getting up and walking around the room at regular intervals. Take long coffee or tea breaks.

Learning to type

This is a contentious point but, if you are going to be serious about writing, it may be a good idea to learn to type. It seems odd to have a very fast and powerful computer coupled to a state-of-the-art word-processing program only to use it to 'hunt and peck' for the keys. There are numerous typing courses available in colleges and as evening classes. There are also some excellent do-it-yourself teaching packages available for use on the computer. One of the best is the interestingly named *Mavis Beacon Teaches Typing* (Erickson 2003). Being able to touch-type and to use all your fingers really does speed up the way you use a computer for writing. It also frees you up to think, not about the keyboard but about the ideas that you have.

> ## RRRRRRapid recap
>
> Check your progress so far by working through each of the following questions.
>
> 1. What is a macro?
> 2. What is a sans serif font?
>
> If you have difficulty with more than one of the questions, read through the section again to refresh your understanding before moving on.

References

Erickson, E. (2003) *Mavis Beacon Teaches Typing*. Southwestern Educational Publishing, Dallas, TX.

Levi, P. (1989) *Other People's Trades*. Abacus, London.

5

Keeping databases

'You must begin by making notes. You may have to make notes for years. . . . When you think of something, when you recall something, put it where it belongs,' he said, 'put it down when you think of it. You may never recapture it quite as vividly the second time.'

F. Scott Fitzgerald

All writers need to keep notes. Some need to keep very specific notes: notes of the books and articles they have written. This chapter is all about how to store information that you need in formats that will enable you to find it again. I admit to working with huge piles of papers. The desk I am sitting at is covered with papers. On the other hand, if I want to find out what books I have read on counselling since 1998, I only have to press a couple of buttons on the computer to find out. The important thing is to organise some of your chaos – even if you don't organise all of it. When preparing to write this chapter I was struck by the number of books on writing that suggest that you carefully organise *all* your information by using elaborate filing systems and methods of cross-reference. A couple of those books' writers were honest enough to admit that 'of course, I don't work that way myself . . . I am much less organised'. This struck me as a bit dishonest. Find a system that suits you and stick to it. Don't get caught up in the interesting but distracting business of building an elaborate database that should allow you to find whatever you want but which takes up so much time in maintenance that it is hardly worth the bother. As before, the keywords are simplicity and structure.

What is a database?

Simply, a database is an organised collection of information. The word tends to be associated with computer programs that file away

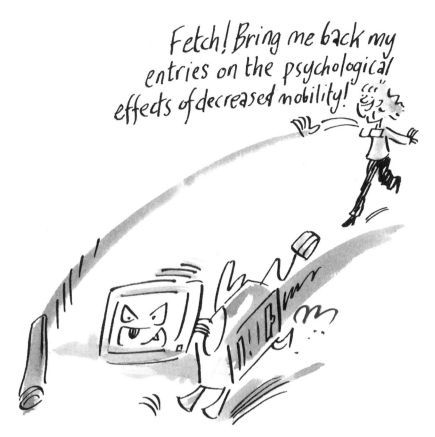

Fetch! Bring me back my entries on the psychological effects of decreased mobility!

A database will store any information you type in and you can retrieve it whenever you want.

information but that limits its use. It is also used to mean a system that allows you to store and retrieve information.

Uses of databases

For the writer, the obvious use of a database is for the storing of bibliographical references. Over the years, I have developed a store of about 1000 such references. Originally, I used a system of cards. Now I use what is called a 'free-form database' program. I will explain the use of both of these methods and others. Also, a writer and researcher can use databases for the following:

- Storing and retrieving interview data
- Storing and retrieving numerical data
- Keeping odd bits of information that are not easily classified

- Storing ideas for papers, articles, research projects and books
- Storing quotable quotes
- Analysing qualitative data
- Storing and retrieving names and addresses
- Keeping track of a project
- Collecting and executing 'to do' lists.

Databases also have lots of other uses and can be used by teachers and practitioners to store details of lectures, case notes and other information that needs to be referred to frequently. Remember, though, if you are going to store personal information about people, you will need to clarify your position regarding the Data Protection Act. You cannot simply store personal information about other people in a computer file. You must first be sure that you are not contravening the Act.

Theory into practice

Learn to access various databases on the Internet. You will find archives of journals, bibliographical databases and files of nursing information, if you know where to look and how to search for them.

Storing bibliographic references

The simplest way of keeping a reference database is by writing the details of the reference on an index card and storing it in a plastic box. Various sorts of card and various sorts of box are available in any stationers. In my experience, most people like buying stationery so this initial part of the process is usually a pleasant one. It is usually preferable to go for the larger 8″ × 5″ cards. These allow you more space for notes.

The card system works like this. You lay out the card as shown in Figure 5.1 (on page 74). Then you file the card alphabetically, using index dividers that you can buy with your box. Later on, when you want to find all your references by a particular author, you simply look up the author's name and find all the references you need.

Another filing method is to keep duplicate cards and use a keyword system. Thus, on the relevant cards, you write COUNSELLING or SOCIAL POLICY and file these together. As long as you know your keywords (and you keep a note of these on a separate card at the front of your box) you can collect together a range of references on a particular topic quickly and easily. Life gets more complicated. What happens with a book like Carl Rogers's *On Becoming a Person*? Do you file it under COUNSELLING or PSYCHOTHERAPY or, perhaps, PSYCHOLOGY?

This is where it soon becomes worth considering using a computerised system. Don't rush too quickly to use one, although I have heard of people setting up reference databases with such heavyweight programs as DBase or Paradox. While it is entirely possible to do this, there may be simpler ways of working.

First of all, though, here is how to complete a reference card. The elements of the card are always the same:

- The name of the surname of the author and her initials
- The year of publication
- The title of the book or paper
- The publisher or name of the journal
- The place of publication or the edition and page numbers of the journal
- Keywords
- Comments.

Figure 5.1 overleaf offers two examples: Figure 5.1a is the reference card for a book and Figure 5.1b shows the reference card for a journal article. You are free, of course, to modify this format to suit yourself. Once you have settled on a format, stick to it.

Using this card format, it is also possible to write direct quotations from the publications straight on to the card for quotation in your essay or article. Two things are important here. First, make sure that you write down the quote exactly as it appears in the book or paper. Make no attempt to tidy up the grammar or spelling. You must leave quotations as they are. Second, make sure you write down the page number. When you use direct quotations in essays and research reports (and you should use them sparingly) you must always state the page number. Thus, a reference to a direct quotation from Figure 5.1a might look like this:

> Used skilfully, gestalt therapy is an arresting, often oblique form of dialogue which involves a wide range of techniques.
>
> Smith 2003: 53

You may not like the grammar nor the language but you must leave the quotation exactly as the author wrote it. As mentioned in Chapter 1, the use of 'sic' should be avoided.

Smith, P.

2003

Learning Interactive Skills: a Reflective Guide for Health Care Professionals, 3rd edition. Butterworth-Heinemann, Oxford.

Keywords: self-awareness, experiential learning, exercises

Comments: Source of activities for learning a range of interpersonal and communication skills. Aimed at nurses but also relevant to other health professionals.

Figure 5.1a *Reference card for a book*

Jones, P.

2004

Spiritual distress and the practical response: theoretical considerations and counselling skills. *Journal of Advanced Health Care* 12: 377–382.

Keywords: Spiritual, counselling, nursing

Comments: A discussion of the problems of 'dispiritedness'. Not necessarily a 'religious' question but definitely a 'spiritual' one. Comments on how counselling skills may be used.

Figure 5.1b *Reference card for a journal article*

As your reference database grows, it will outgrow the plastic container you spent so much time choosing. You then have a number of choices:

- Buy another plastic container and begin to fill that up
- Buy a filing drawer: this will take you years to fill up
- Consider computerising your system.

Key points **Top tips**

- Be accurate in recording bibliographical references: author, date, title, publisher, place of publication
- Use a computerised database system if at all possible
- Back up your database regularly
- 'Weed' your database every six months and remove references that you really do not need.

Computer databases

Databases for computers come in two types: the fixed-form database and the free-form sort. I will discuss both as both have their advantages and disadvantages.

The fixed-form database

First, some definitions. A form, in database jargon, is a single record. Thus an entry containing all the details of one book is called a form. Each form contains a number of fields. A field is a discrete unit of information. Thus the place where you put the author's name is a field. So is the place where you put the date. So is the place where you put the title, and so on.

With a fixed-form database, you have to work out a number of things before you start to file away your references. First, you need to know how many fields you will have. Then, you need to know the maximum length of any given field. For example, a simple reference database might have the following fields (and I have numbered them so that you can see at a glance how many fields there are):

1. Surname and initials of author
2. Year of publication
3. Title
4. Publisher and place of publication
5. Keywords
6. Comments.

For all these fields, you will need to consider the length of the field. You have to know this sort of information in advance of entering data. There is a problem here. It is tempting, at first, to play safe and make the fields as long as possible – just in case you get an author with a triple-barrelled name or a title that goes on forever. On the other hand, if you do this, you are likely to take up a lot of space on your hard disk. Also, databases with long fields take a long time to 'search' (or look up) and, with some databases, the display on the screen may be affected by long fields. You need to think carefully, then, about a reasonable length for each field. Here are some values that I have found useful. The numbers in each case refer to the number of characters that can be used in a field. A character is a number, figure or space.

1. Author (100)
2. Date (4)

3. Title (250)

4. Publisher (200)

5. Keywords (50)

6. Comments (250).

Why 250 for the longer fields? Many databases have an upper limit of 250 characters per field.

When you are designing your database, you may want to add additional fields. Here are some that you might want to consider:

7. Location (library, home, work, named person)

8. Date of this entry

9. Lent to

and so on.

Key points **Top tips**

- Be careful – do not make your database system too complicated
- Simplicity is important
- If you make your database lengthy and complicated you will find yourself skipping many of the fields and end up with an incomplete database
- As a rule, only record the information that you are going to need in the future.

Once you have settled on the layout, the fields and the field lengths, you are stuck with that format. While it is possible to change the format at a later date, it can be difficult. The best thing to do is to have a few trial runs at making database layouts. Then choose the one that looks and feels best.

Once you have worked out the layout of your forms and fields, you can begin to enter the data. You can put the references in any order, for the program can order all your cards afterwards. Mostly, you will want them indexed alphabetically by author but you can choose other permutations. Also, you can ask the database to call up all the entries that contain a particular keyword. Thus, you can call up all the entries that contain the keyword COUNSELLING and browse through all the references that you have collected on that topic. Further, you can narrow your search, if you have a lot of references on a particular topic. If, for example, you have hundreds of references on GROUPS, you may want to limit your search to GROUPS, THERAPY. The database program will then call up only those references that are to do with group therapy rather than just groups.

Also, you might want to call up all a particular author's works on a particular subject. An example of this would be calling up everything that you have by Carl Rogers on client-centred counselling. This would mean that the program would ignore anything that Rogers had written (and you had collected) on topics such as humanistic psychology or student-centred learning. The database program can be a very flexible way of working with your reference collection. I know that I would be very reluctant to go back to a card system. As always, back-up your database files. If your hard disk crashes, it is likely that you will have lost all your hard-found references.

Examples of fixed-form database programs

There are numerous commercial programs on the market. The larger ones include the following.

- Access: this is a large and powerful database program from Microsoft. It is, however, also one of the easiest to use. I used to use it for storing bibliographical references and still use it, at work, to store student records.

- Paradox: powerful and yet easy to use: hence the name. The two features do not usually go hand in hand. I know a number of people who use this database as a referencing system.

○━┓ Keywords

Querying the database
Looking something up

These programs vary in price and complexity. Remember that you ideally want something that is simple to use and to '**query the database**'.

You may well find that one of the shareware programs is just what you need. The concept of shareware is discussed in Chapter 3 on page 57.

Free-form databases

The free-form database does not use concepts such as fields and field length. With the free-form database, you simply open up a form, type in whatever it is you want to save, save the form and that is it. To look up an item of saved information, you simply key in one or two words that you know are in the form that you saved and the form comes on the screen. You are not limited by the format in which you enter data. You can put the author's name, followed by the title, followed by the date or you can start with a quotation and follow it with the bibliographic reference. The format really does not matter. All that matters is that you remember a word or two that occurs in the form that you have written. The free-form database program is rather like being able to collect together all sorts of different notes and pieces of paper and then being able to pull out the relevant ones whenever you want. I find the free-form approach much more liberating for storing bibliographic details. Figure 5.2 shows two examples of two forms from a free-form system. Note that both are in a very different format but that both can happily co-exist in the same database.

Davies, P. 2004 Counselling Skills for Carers: 2nd edition: Nelson Thornes, Cheltenham.

This contains a number of chapters on counselling theory and reviews different approaches to counselling. It does not only address client-centred counselling but considers other types too.

I have lent my copy of this to David Jones. Remember to ring him about this.

His address is:
David Jones,
35 Blakemore Cottages
Denfield
Herts CF4 3RT

Also, consider the books by Rogers when it comes to writing up the counselling research project.

Keywords: Counselling, humanistic psychology, psychoanalysis, behavioural psychology

This is a list of some of the books on COUNSELLING that may be helpful. Remember to look in Cardiff Central Library, too. They have a lot of useful books.

Baruth, L.G. 1987 An Introduction to the Counselling Profession: Prentice Hall, Englewood Cliffs, New Jersey
Bolger, A.W. (ed 1982E) Counselling in Britain: a reader: Batsford Academic, London
Dryden, W., Charles-Edwards and Woolfe, R. 1989 Handbook of Counselling in Britain Routledge

Figure 5.2 *Examples of forms from a free-form system*

Maintaining your database

Whether you use the fixed-form database or the free-form database, a few basic rules apply to maintenance.

Key points Top tips

- Always make sure you back-up your database files to floppies once you have finished entering new data

- Get to know the program well. Learn how to index and how to transfer data from your database to your word-processing program and *vice versa*

- Be careful to plan your database layout before you begin to use it. The best place to start is with pen and paper. Try a few layouts on paper before you experiment with the program itself

- Databases are personal things, rather in the way that word-processing programs are. Do not use a particular one just because someone has recommended it to you

- Try to review a few before making a final decision and then be prepared to change your mind.

Initially, I worked with a word-processing file full of references. This was a straightforward system until the file got rather large. With this system, you simply list your references, in alphabetical order, in an ordinary word-processing file, like this:

Bradbury, R. (1990) *Zen in the Art of Writing: Essays on creativity: Joshua Odell editions*. Capra Press, Santa Barbara, California.

Fitzgerald, F.S. Afternoon of an author. In: Phillips L.W. (1985) *F. Scott Fitzgerald on Writing*. Scribner, New York.

Gunning, R. (1968) *The Technique of Clear Writing*, 2nd edn. McGraw-Hill, London.

Jourard, S. (1971) *Self-disclosure: An experimental analysis of the transparent self*. Wiley, New York.

Larson, M. (1986) *Literary Agents: How to get and work with the right one for you*. Writer's Digest Books, Cincinnati, Ohio.

Wright Mills, C. (1959) *The Sociological Imagination*. Oxford University Press, Oxford.

You are then free to cut and paste references into papers and articles that you write. If your word processor has an automatic sorting function, you can enter the references into the file in any order. Then you ask the word processor to sort, alphabetically.

I used this system for a couple of years. I would call up the reference file every time I wrote a paper and kept it on the 'second screen'. That meant that I could easily switch between the paper I was writing and the reference file. Once this file became too big, I looked at a variety of simple database programs and finally settled on Idealist.

Data Protection Act

If you keep details about other people on disk, you must notify this under the Data Protection Act 1998. There are eight general principles behind the Act. These are:

- Personal data must be collected and used fairly without deceiving those concerned
- Any personal data kept must be notified under the Act
- If you are going to pass on personal data to other people you must state this when you notify under the Data Protection Act
- You should not keep more personal data than you need
- You have to try to make sure that personal data is accurate and up to date
- You should not keep personal data for longer than you need to
- If you hold personal data about somebody, they have the right to know what it is and to check that it is accurate
- You have to try to make sure that personal data is not changed, destroyed or disclosed without authorisation.

Notification of your personal data store can be done on-line and costs approximately £35 a year. The information you will require to supply includes the following:

- The personal data you are recording
- What you use the data for
- Where you get this information from
- Whom you may want to disclose it to
- Any overseas countries to which you may want to send the information.

You do not have to notify under the Act if you are merely keeping a personal address book, nor do you have to register if you keep a list of the members of a club or society. You should check with your employers whether or not you are covered by the Act if you use your own database systems to record details of students on courses. You must consider too whether or not you need to undertake notification if you record personal details about people for a research project. Clearly, you do not have to register in order to maintain databases of non-personal details such as bibliographies.

*ᵃᴿᴿᴿᴿ***Rapid recap**

Check your progress so far by working through both the following questions.

1. List three reasons why a writer should keep a database.
2. What are the six fields recommended for a simple reference database?

If you have difficulty with either of the questions, read through the section again to refresh your understanding before moving on.

References

Smith, P. (2003) *Learning Interactive Skills: A reflective guide for health care professionals*, 3rd edn. Butterworth-Heinemann, Oxford.

Educational writing

To write simply is as difficult as to be good.

Somerset Maugham

Most lecturers and educationalists have to write. But, increasingly, students also have to give presentations, feedback to their colleagues and teach other groups. For university and college lecturers, writing is sometimes part of the job, as it is for students. Increasingly, too, students are encouraged to contribute articles and books as part of their contribution to the literature. Chapters 9 and 10 of this book are concerned specifically with writing articles and books. The aim of this chapter is to explore elements of writing as it applies to preparing educational materials, although if you're a new student you will find it useful too.

The sort of writing that has to be done by a teacher or lecturer will include the following:

- Preparation of overhead transparencies
- Preparation of handouts
- Writing of course material
- Writing of curriculum documents
- Preparing notes for a presentation or conference
- Writing letters, memos and faxes
- Sending e-mail messages.

Overhead transparencies

Overhead transparencies (OHTs) are widely used by teachers and lecturers. They are a means of conveying headings and specific information to large groups of people. They also take the spotlight off the teacher or lecturer and allow her to concentrate on good delivery.

These days, most laser printers or photocopiers can produce print on to acetate sheets. If your laser or dot matrix printer cannot, your photocopier is likely to. Now you have no excuse for scrappy, handwritten OHTs. Instead, you can print out single sheets of text, which you then photocopy on to acetates, making enlargements as necessary.

Key points Top tips

Certain key principles apply to the preparation of material for OHTs:

- Keep them simple
- Use clear and straightforward graphics to illustrate a point, where possible
- Use only one or two fonts – no more
- Use only a few lines per sheet.

I once sat through the most boring lecture I can remember. The lecturer used a single sheet, which was covered in writing. She slowly revealed a single line of text and took about 10 minutes to talk through each item. You knew how much longer the lecture had to run by the amount she still had to reveal. The lecture seemed to go on for ever.

Although the revelation technique is widely taught as a method of working through OHTs, I think that it has one big disadvantage. It reminds the students of how much is to come. Better, I think, to use one or two straightforward acetates that you reveal completely and then talk through. Do not have too many sheets. Almost as daunting as the sheet covered in writing that is gradually revealed is the ominous looking pile of acetates next to the projector that you know the lecturer is going to get through, come what may. Again, keep it short and simple. Use illustrations wherever possible. Try to make your presentations as professional as possible.

Some lecturers like to use slides. Again, make full use of these by taking photographs and showing these, interspersed with single slides containing words. Usually, slides with writing on have a blue background with white lettering. Try, if you can, to ring the changes and have different-coloured backgrounds. Also, consider combining either two slide projectors and two screens or the overhead projector (OHP) and a slide machine. I have seen joint use of these contribute to a very effective presentation.

Don't overuse slides. Use perhaps five or six. Any more and the presentation gets to be reminiscent of those awful evenings that you sometimes get invited to when a friend shows her holiday slides or photos. Most people overestimate other people's interest in a particular topic. Make sure, too, that your slides are of the highest quality and that all are set in the right position in the slide projector.

Nothing upsets the lecturer and amuses an audience quite as much as an upside-down slide. When you show the slide, after a quick glance to see that it is both up the right way and also the right slide, talk to the audience and not to the slide. Allow people a little time to stare at the slide and do not offer any important information during the first 30 seconds of slide display. Try, if you can, to use the slides and OHP material to surprise and delight the audience. Boring slides can do nothing to enhance and audience and nothing to improve the quality of your presentation.

Theory into practice

If you have to make a presentation of your work at university, consider offering to do something similar in the ward or community setting in which you next work. In this way, you can share your knowledge and information with your colleagues who may not be undertaking a course like yours.

Use a graphics program to produce clear printed sheets, perhaps containing three or four lines, in a single font.

Whatever you do, make sure that all your visual aids are professionally prepared. Become familiar with what your graphics program can do and use it minimally. That is to say that you should not become over ambitious. You can always tell the amateur who has just acquired a graphics package: her OHTs are covered with familiar symbols from well-known graphics programs. Often, butterflies, balloons and buildings feature strongly in such presentations.

Increasingly, people are working directly from the slides made on their computer to a projector. This usually means that a laptop computer is plugged straight into the projector and the images from the computer program are projected on to a screen. As long as the place at which a presentation is being made has the projector, this is often the easiest thing to do. Increasingly, too, projectors are becoming smaller and it is possible to travel with both the laptop *and* the projector to the site of the presentation.

Preparation of handouts

Many of the principles of OHT preparation apply to handouts. Keep them simple and use only one or two fonts in their preparation. Make sure that all photocopies are clearly printed and completely readable.

Conventional teaching wisdom has it that you should not give out handouts during a lecture but at the end. This is to stop the distraction of the pile of papers being handed round the room. It is also to stop people reading the handouts instead of listening to you. In practice, I find it useful to do one-page handouts that contain broad headings and to give those out. If these pages are clearly numbered, they remove the need for students to continually jot down notes as you are speaking and the students have a permanent *aide-mémoire* of your lecture. Again, if you prepare such handouts carefully and professionally, it reflects well on you as a lecturer. Scrappy or unclear handouts also reflect on you.

Go easy with book lists. The temptation is to hand out three- or four-page lists of books. Few people read through such lists and I suspect that few lecturers have read all the books on their lists. Anyone, really, can compile huge bibliographies fairly easily. Instead, consider one-page book lists containing perhaps six or seven titles that constitute essential reading. Then offer yourself as a resource for the keen student who wants advice about further reading.

Key points | **Top tips**

- Rehearse your presentation and time it
- Keep presentations simple
- A blue background with white or yellow lettering, on acetates and presentations, is often easiest to read.

Preparing notes

Some students now give papers at conferences. Many are terrified at the thought and many are not very good at it because they do not prepare sufficiently.

To read from notes or not to? Not to, as a rule. If at all possible, avoid reading directly from a script or straight from notes. If you can read what you have to say, so can your audience. If all you are doing is standing up and reading what you would normally publish in a journal, do the latter. Go away and write your journal paper. While you may not want to do without notes altogether (and few do), you want to try to keep your notes to key issues and an overall outline structure.

The most frequently used method of using notes at a presentation is that of holding a bunch of index cards in your hand, each of which contains notes linked to one of your three or four points. These have advantages and disadvantages. The advantages are that they are easy to hold and to refer to. You can hold your hands up fairly high and this tends to encourage you to speak out to your audience rather than down to your notes. On the other hand, small cards can be dropped. Once dropped, you have the unenviable (but fascinating to the audience in a morbid sort of way) task of picking them up and rearranging them. Just in case, it is best to number your cards with fairly large numbers so that your nervous hands can reorder them in a crisis.

It is usually best to link your cards with your visual presentations. As noted in the next section, backing up what you say with things that the audience can look at pays distinct dividends. Usually, you can link one card with one visual aid. In this way, you don't have to carry out too many operations at once. Be sure, though, to clearly number both your cards and your visual aids. Visual aids can also be dropped or get out of order. If both the card and the aid bear the same number, you are less likely to run into problems.

The alternative to cards is to use a computer-generated set of notes. If you use this method, you need to have them typed with double spacing, so that you can read them easily as you glance down. Also, it is useful to make full use of coloured 'outlining' pens. Careful colour coding can show you where you are in relation to your main three or four points: each point can be outlined in a different colour and that colour code can be carried through to your visual aids. The big disadvantage of typed sheets is that you are likely to get carried away with looking at them.

There is some comfort to be had from holding a large bunch of papers. Often, that comfort takes over and the speaker using them stares down at them throughout the presentation, sometimes from fear of losing the place. Think, too, about whether or not you staple the sheets together. The advantage of this approach is that you can hold the whole set of pages together with less fear of dropping them. On the other hand, if you find yourself with a large lectern in front of you, unstapled sheets can more easily be turned over. I have been known to adopt the 'belt and braces' approach and take two sets of notes with me to a conference, one stapled and the other not.

If your confidence really leaves you and you decide that you must read from notes, consider the way that you write out those notes. Rather than just typing out a 'script', write out what you say in the way that you say it. Figure 6.1 illustrates this. The piece is laid out in such a way that it makes it very clear where you pause and where you take a breath. The idea is that each line contains one phrase. Work carefully through your notes and break them up in this way.

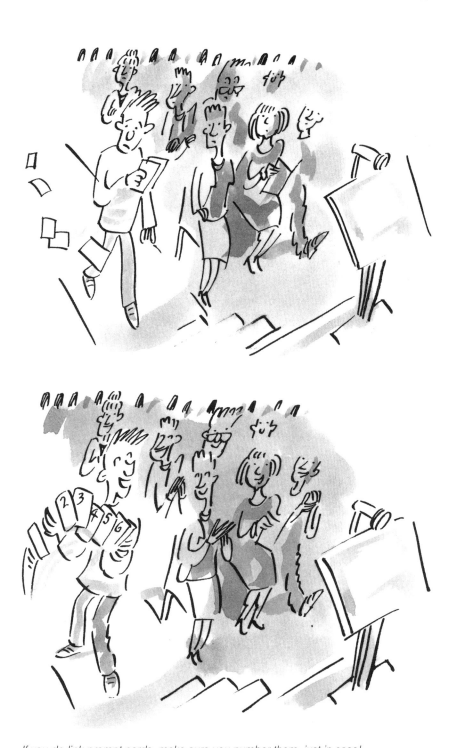

If you do link prompt cards, make sure you number them, just in case!

Conference Paper: Change and the Health Professional

1. Many health professionals are having to think carefully about how change is affecting their organisation.
2. Many are experiencing anxiety about the rate of change.
3. Writers on the topic are not always helpful here.
4. All seem to stress that change is accelerating.
5. This morning, I want to challenge that view.
6. The question is: Is the rate of change really increasing?
7. Think about your own workplace.
8. What changes have you seen?
9. Major ones?
10. Or have you experienced a slow trickle of minor changes?
11. If change is occurring, what difference does it make?
12. People as resilient and able to cope.
13. Defence mechanisms.
14. What the research tells us.
15. Concluding comments.

Figure 6.1 *Example of notes for a conference paper*

This will save you 'fluffing' lines and save you having to re-read what you have said. It must be stressed, however, that reading direct from a paper is the last resort. If you can, avoid it.

One of the best ways of preparing this sort of paper is on a computer, using a word-processing program. It is possible, in some programs, to set up 'macros' or short-hand routines that operate 'sentence-busting' functions. Such macros split the whole of your paper up into sentences and put each sentence on a separate line. WordPerfect is one such program. It is possible, with this program, not only to sentence-bust but also to reverse the process and put the paper back together again. In this way, you are able to prepare the paper that you use for your presentation and the more usual copies of the paper for wider distribution. Be careful, though: splitting the paper into sentences is not all that is involved. You also need to go through the piece and underline or accent certain words so that you know exactly when to emphasise your points. Notice, too, that the piece in Figure 6.1 is not strictly grammatical.

You may want to consider the use of rhetorical questions that 'sound' right when you speak but would not normally be acceptable in a written paper. Again, this is further fuel for the argument that you should try to avoid reading directly from a script. On the other hand, if you are giving a lot of very detailed information and that information must be exactly right, then reading may be your only option. Consider, for example, newsreaders on the television. No one would expect them to extemporise with the help of cue cards.

Curriculum vitae

The other sort of educational writing that many students have to write or advise other people about is writing a curriculum vitae. The curriculum vitae is just that: a 'life curriculum' or description of your life to date. Think carefully about what you put in it. It is usually a good idea to keep a copy of your CV in your possession at all times and to update it regularly. That way, when you apply for a job, there is no problem in remembering what you have and have not done. If you use a computer, it is useful to keep your CV as a word-processing file and to add to the file as new things happen to you. You may want to keep a 'short version' that summarises the essential parts of your personal history, as well as the full version. The short version can be a useful aid to filling in application forms and may be asked for during applications for jobs, grants or scholarships. It is also possible to write macros in a word-processing program to recall, quickly, your prepared CV.

CVs typically cover the following subject areas:

- Name
- Address
- Work address
- Date of birth
- Age
- Marital status
- Place of birth
- Nationality
- Current post
- Secondary, professional and higher education
- Other professional training (short courses, management courses, etc.)
- Professional employment
- Summary of responsibilities in present post
- Committee membership
- Other professional activities (membership of unions, clubs, associations, editorial boards, external examining, etc.)

- Other activities (governorship of schools, membership of other organisations, etc.)
- Miscellaneous section (driving licence, word-processing skills, etc.)
- Research
- Conference papers
- Publications (books, chapters in books, articles in refereed journals, articles in other journals).

You might not use all these headings nor will they all be appropriate to everyone's CV but you should aim at making your CV as comprehensive as possible. Make sure that all the dates are correct and that the spelling and layout are appropriate. At the end of the CV it is sometimes correct to include the names and addresses of two or three people who will write references for you. Make sure that you ask those people's permission to quote their names before you do so.

Make sure that you spend some time on the layout of your CV. Too many people spoil an otherwise excellent CV by one or other of two extremes. Some spoil the document by overuse of a desktop publishing program. Such people use coloured paper, lots of different-sized fonts and full use of banner headlines and so forth. They make their CV look more like a parish newsletter than a serious document of their lives. At the other extreme, some people type their CV on a battered typewriter with an old ribbon and an uneven typeface. Try for something in the middle. Laser print your CV but use only standard headings and subheadings. Use white paper only and try, above all things, to make the document look business-like. It is, after all, a sales document.

Note that, nowadays, many word processors are supplied with a CV template or a method of formatting a CV to make it look professional and to standardise the layout.

Another sort of CV is one that concentrates on your achievements. In this type, you write out your life history in terms of your educational and professional posts and under each one you list the things that you achieved. An example of such an entry might be the following:

Lecturer in Health Visiting, University of Blackheath: 1999–2001. During this period, I was course leader for the health visiting course. I rewrote the curriculum, advised on promotion and advertising and was able to recruit three times the number of students in 2000 than in the previous year.

Writing letters, memos, faxes and e-mails

Most students have to send a variety of letters, faxes and e-mails. Most people soon get the hang of wording such documents and, once again, the key features of simplicity and structure apply. There are also some conventions for laying out such documents. Figures 6.2, 6.3 and 6.4 show the conventional layout for letters, memos and faxes.

Fashions in layout change. Currently, it is popular to use the 'block' paragraph layout for paragraphs in letters, memos and faxes. Also, it is usual to layout text 'ranged left'. That is to say that headings, addresses and so forth are lined up against the left margin rather than centred on the page or ranged to the right.

Bear in mind that if you are using a modern word-processing program you can usually set up a template or a macro that will allow you to call up a 'blank' letter, memo or fax page and then simply 'fill in the blanks'. This approach is not only economical of time but it also helps you to maintain a consistent corporate image.

Scotfield University College

23–45 Anderson Road

Scotfield

Surrey

SC1 N4T

Phone: 01243–342523

24th May 2003

Dr Sarah Jones

56 Petersfield Road

Langley

South Glamorgan

CF5 43L

Dear Sarah

Stress Reduction Teaching

Thank you for your recent letter. I am glad that you were able to use the activities that I suggested. I have found them particularly useful when teaching small groups.

I hope that we will be able to keep in touch about these approaches to helping people with stress. I look forward to hearing from you again.

With best wishes,

Yours sincerely,

Dr Susan Brownloe

Director of Health Care Studies

Figure 6.2 *Layout of a letter*

MEMO

To: Jane Johnson, Senior Health Lecturer, University College

From: Peter Barker, Lecturer, School of Occupational Therapy, University College

Date: 23.4.03

Re: Course Evaluation

Thank you for sending me the evaluation questionnaires. I have made copies of them and circulated them to my colleagues. Once I have used the questionnaires with the student group, I will collate the findings and send them to you.

Figure 6.3 *Layout of a memo*

Scotfield University College
23–45 Anderson Road
Scotfield
Surrey
SC1 N4T

Fax Cover Sheet

DATE:	2 December 2003	TIME:	15:30
TO:	Mr P. Jones	PHONE:	01243–342523
	Anderson Health College	FAX:	01243–353243
FROM:	Dr A. Davies	PHONE:	01453–234525
	Scotfield University College	FAX:	01453–465463
RE:	Interdisciplinary Health Teaching		
CC:	Mrs J. Arthurs, Personal Assistant		

Number of pages including cover sheet: 1

Thank you for the curriculum document. I will take it to the curriculum planning committee in this college this afternoon. I will then contact you again, with further details of the next stage, directly after the meeting.

This is the name and address that you need in order to purchase copies of the open learning materials that we discussed:

Peter Sharpe
Abacus Open Learning College
34 London Road
Abingail
Wiltshire WV4 5D6

Phone: 01442–564364

Figure 6.4 *Layout of a fax*

Note that memos don't usually need to be signed by the sender and may not need an envelope if they are being sent through an internal postal system. As a rule, they should be kept short: you want them to be *read*.

When writing faxes, it is often better to use a sans serif font for the body text of the fax – as shown in Figure 6.4. A sans serif font tends to 'copy' better when passed through the two fax machines. Note that you can either use a cover page that is blank – except for the details of the person sending it and the person receiving it – as the first page of your fax or you can write your message straight on to the first page of the fax. It is often preferable to use a 'blank' cover page if you know that your fax contains sensitive information of if you know that it may lie in a pile at the organisation to whom you are sending it. In these cases, the cover page serves to cover up the information contained in your fax.

As with all writing, it is important to make sure that memos, letters and faxes are clear and make use of simple language. The days of letters being written in a peculiar 'officialese' are largely over but it is still possible to find people writing regularly, 'Please find enclosed a copy of the report' instead of the more straightforward, 'Here is a copy of the report'.

E-mail

The style of writing when sending and responding to e-mail is much less formal than is the case with letters, memos and faxes. E-mail communication is almost like a conversation. It is quite acceptable to write in note form when responding to e-mail. An example of a continuing 'correspondence' might look like the example in Figure 6.5. It should be noted that new messages on the e-mail will be prefaced by details of the sender, their e-mail address and the route by which the e-mail message travelled. These details are omitted in Figure 6.5. They can run to many lines of screen print-out.

In summary, all educational writing is a form of communication. It is also part of the educational process. You should spend time planning how you will use printed matter. After all, it is the format that most people use to learn a lot of what they know. Students will spend hours reading books and journal articles. If you're a lecturer, don't insult them by giving them poorly prepared handouts or course material. Do not upset them by offering them ill-prepared OHTs during your lectures. Besides, planning and designing this sort of material can be interesting in and of itself. Read more about layout

15 April 2004 08:48

Dear Peter,

Do you have any details of the work of Peters and Davies on learning styles? I believe they developed a learning styles inventory some years ago but I can't find it.

Regards,
David French,
University of West London

15 April 2004 09:30

Dear David,

I found your learning styles inventory. It was published in a journal that only has a small circulation and I can understand why you missed it. Here is the reference:

Peters, D.A. and Davies, P. 1995 Measuring How People Learn: is it possible? *New England Health Care Journal, 3, 4, 23–56.*

A colleague in Florida has used the inventory. Do you want me to get her to contact you?

Regards,
Peter Zander,
University of Chicago.

16 April 2004 10:05

Dear Peter,

Thanks for the reference – I have tracked down the paper. That was useful. Yes, I would be delighted to hear from your colleague in Florida. Thanks again.

Regards,
David

18 April 2004 08:16

Dear David French,

Peter Zander at the University of Chicago asked me to contact you. I hear that you are interested in using the Peters and Davies' learning styles inventory. I have used it with four groups of between 100–150 students and will send you a summary of my findings. Perhaps we could do some collaborative research on this?

Regards,
Sally Henderson,
Lecturer in Health Care Studies,
University of Southern Florida,
E-mail address sallyh@fla.edu

Figure 6.5 *Example of e-mail dialogue*

and printing. Particularly, learn the basic rules of layout and make them second nature. Then your own printed work will always look professional and will be appreciated by your students and your colleagues.

RRRRRRapid recap

Check your progress so far by working through both the following questions.

1. What does OHT stand for?

2. List three ways of preparing your notes for giving a presentation.

If you have difficulty with either of the questions, read through the section again to refresh your understanding before moving on.

Writing essays

> Clear writers, like clear fountains, do not seem so deep as they are; the turbid look the most profound.
>
> Walter Savage Landor

If you are doing a course of some kind that lasts longer than a week, you are likely to have to write essays. Essays are an almost universal form of assessment. While there are numerous titles for essays, there are some simple rules about writing that can be learned fairly easily. The aim of this chapter is to make your essay writing easier. It has to be said, though, that some people like writing and write easily while others struggle to put pen to paper or fingers to keyboard. Whether you find it pleasure or pain, the keynote, once again, is structure. If you can get the structure right you are likely to find the writing easier. This applies if this is your first or 31st essay. No one should sit down and begin to write the first line of an essay without prior planning.

The planning stages of an essay are as follows:

- Reading the question
- Underlining key words
- Brainstorming
- Writing the essay outline
- Collecting information.

Reading the question

This would seem to be a straightforward requirement. Many people tend to write the essay they think should be written rather than the one that is asked for. Some people have a 'standard' essay that is almost automatically written whenever key words are seen. For example, an essay about counselling skills in helping bereaved people may cause some people to write everything they know about counselling. This is not the point at all. It is vital to answer the question. This can only happen if you read the question carefully and re-read it.

Underlining the key words

Once you have read the question, underline the key words. This is not as simple as it sounds. Some people find when they first do this that they underline almost all the words in the essay title. Here is a sample question to work on:

> Critically evaluate the use of therapy groups in a specific health-care setting.

Read through the title two or three times and then underline the key words. The underlining that I did was as follows:

> <u>Critically evaluate</u> the use of <u>therapy groups</u> in a <u>specific health-care setting</u>.

Now consider what the essay is asking you to do. First, you are asked to *critically evaluate* something. Not describe it. Not define it but critically evaluate it. Think carefully about what that means. Then, you are given the subject of that critical evaluation: *therapy groups*. This means that you have to be clear about what therapy groups might be and you will need to say this in your essay. Finally, you are asked to do all of this within a *specific health-care setting*. As no other details are given, it can be taken as read that you can choose the health-care setting. Make sure that you do. Make sure that you tell the reader what setting you have chosen. All of this must happen before you move on to the next stage of brainstorming.

Over to you

Underline what you consider to be the key words in the following essay titles:

- Assess the importance of infection control for health-care professionals
- Analyse the psychological effects of a critical care environment on the patients within these areas
- Compare the role of spirituality in two different clinical settings.

---**Keywords**

Analyse
To examine in depth the elements of . . .

Assess
To estimate, in a balanced way, the value and importance of . . .

Compare
To look for similarities and differences between . . ., perhaps reaching a conclusion as to which is preferable

In the last activity were you clear about the different expectations for these essays suggested by the terms **assess**, **analyse** and **compare**? It is important that you have a clear understanding of the keywords.

Brainstorming

Most people are fairly familiar with the process of brainstorming and it is only briefly described here. It is noteworthy that, while brainstorming tends to be taught in UK schools and colleges, formal outlining of essays does not. In Canada and the USA, outlining is taught at junior school level. Perhaps we need to give it more attention in the UK. It can make all the difference in essay writing.

Brainstorming involves giving the imagination free rein around the topic in hand. Having read the question and having identified what the question is about, the brainstorming phase is concerned with your jotting down on a piece of paper all the words or associations that you can think of related to the question. These should be written down in any order and *everything* is permitted. Make no attempt to filter out any words of phrases and do not work at 'ordering' at this stage. The dafter ideas often spark off useful ones. Here is an example of some of the things that I 'brainstormed' around the previously given essay title:

- Group therapy
- Gestalt therapy
- Group facilitation
- Health-care setting: acute psychiatric unit
- Psychiatrist
- Psychologist
- Who runs the group?
- Research into groups?
- Do groups work?
- My wife doesn't like groups much
- Types of group facilitation
- Does therapy work?
- J. Masson: *Beyond Therapy*
- References for this essay?
- I like group work
- I like running groups
- I don't enjoy being a member so much

- Are groups about power?
- How do you evaluate groups?
- What is a group?
- Offer clear definitions at the start of your essay
- Who is this essay for?
- Groups or counselling: which is best?
- Training.

This brainstorming process should carry on for as long as you can still make associations around the title of the essay. The process may last for 5 minutes or it may last for 15. Do not leave any thoughts out and allow yourself to muse a little.

Next, work through the list and cross out any obviously inappropriate words or phrases. In the above list, I think I would cross out 'I don't like being a member so much' and 'Groups or counselling: which is best?'. Both have relevance for the essay in that they reminded me about my own bias in group work and about counselling – a related but not directly relevant issue. The latter point also reminded me of a book by Richard Nelson Jones in which he discusses 'group counselling'. However, neither of those two phrases seem directly related to the topic in hand.

The next stage is to group together the various issues into some sort of order. This is often best done under a series of headings. The headings that seem to emerge from the above list would include:

- The context (the setting)
- Definitions
- Problems of evaluation
- Issues in running therapy groups.

From this initial grouping together, the structure of a possible essay begins to emerge and it is possible to begin to draw up an outline. An outline is what it says: the headings and subheadings of your essay. An outline for the above essay might look like this:

1. **Introduction**
   a. What this essay is about
2. **Definitions**
   a. Therapy groups
   b. Health-care setting
   c. Evaluation
3. **Health-care setting**
   a. Acute psychiatric unit
   b. Brief description
   c. Uses of therapy groups in this setting

4. Evaluating groups

    a.   Short review of the research

    b.   Methods of evaluating groups

5. Critical issues

    a.   Lack of specific research

    b.   Difficulty in deciding whether or not group work is effective in psychiatry

    c.   Tendency of some practitioners to prefer group work

6. Summary

    a.   Summing up: review of the main points

    b.   Directions for future work

    c.   Conclusions.

7. References

Over to you

Try brainstorming around the question: 'Explore the psychological effects of incontinence on a patient'.

Once the outline is completed, it is important to check back to the question and to the brainstorming to check that the outline is for an essay that answers the question. Read through the above outline and be critical of it yourself. Is it likely to answer the question? Does it look as though key issues may be left out? How does it compare to an essay that *you* might write on the topic? Essays are bound to reflect the view of the person who writes them. They will also vary in 'depth' according to the course they are being written for. You would not necessarily expect a detailed, analytical and researched-based paper on a pre-training course. You would expect such a paper on a masters degree course.

Make sure that you are writing the right sort of essay for the course you are working on. If you are unsure of the level, ask to see an example essay. Most lecturers are able to show you something of this sort if they are pushed, although some are hedgy about the issue.

Theory into practice

Consider offering copies of your marked essays to go in a file on the ward or in the community setting in which you work. This will further help colleagues to keep up to date.

Collecting information

Using the outline, you can collect all the information you need to write your essay. Often, this will involve the library. It will mean your collecting 'references': details of books and papers related to the topic in your essay. You can get this information in a number of ways. The following is a list of some of these:

- By browsing through the library shelves. This can be time-consuming but can turn up some surprises. It can produce serendipitous findings: surprising and pleasant. It can also waste a lot of time.
- By working through the books that you already have on the topic and referring to the books that have been used by the writer. If you were writing an essay on writing, for example, you could turn to the bibliography section of this book to find more references.
- By using library bibliographies. These are large volumes in the library that list all recent publications in a given field. They often list an abstract of a particular book or paper, too.
- By using CD-ROM. This is a compact disk, computerised system of bibliographic storage. It is the most efficient way of finding references. You can print out lists of the references you need, filter huge lists of references down to more specific lists. You can also download your reference lists on to floppy disk for use later on.

Once you have got your references together, you need to record them in the format described in the earlier chapter. Then, you need to find the books and papers and read them.

Key points *Top tips*

- Plan and outline your essay
- Write simply, clearly and do not try to be 'clever' when you write
- Check your references, spelling and grammar
- Check that you are within the word limit required.

Writing the essay

All that remains is to write the essay. Using the outline, work through each of the headings and follow the plan. Make sure that you only write about the issues under the particular heading. Be careful that you do not get carried away and write everything down under one heading.

Use the headings from your proposal as headings in the essay. Although opinions differ about whether or not headings should be used in essays, the trend towards their use seems to have increased. On the whole, they tend to lend structure to the essay and offer 'signposts' to the reader. More traditional lecturers may ask that you avoid using them.

Also a matter of debate is whether or not you should highlight the main points of your essay in your introduction. An example of such an introduction might be:

> Evaluation of any psychological therapy is likely to be difficult. The question of the efficacy of group therapy has been the subject of considerable debate but not of very much research. This paper opens with definitions of the terms used in it. The health-care setting is then defined. The paper continues with a critical debate of the issue of evaluating group therapy in that context.

Despite the rather prosaic tone of this opening paragraph, it does help to guide the reader to what is going to be in the essay. Likewise, a similar paragraph at the end of the essay helps to draw together the main threads and to highlight the important issues. Some, however, feel that both are redundant. Some academics prefer a more direct style that entails getting straight into the meat of the essay. Find out from the person who has set your essay which approach applies.

References

Use references carefully in your essay. Never use them just to impress. In a sense, of course, this is a slightly pompous statement: you are *trying* to impress when you write your essay. References, though, should indicate that you are aware of the source of particular ideas, thoughts, research and so forth. You should not use them as cake decorations to brighten up your essay. Nor should you quote directly from text unless you feel that you cannot possibly paraphrase what the other writer has written. Direct quotations should be gems. Also, it is best to gather your references together at the ends of sentences rather than scattering them throughout. Consider, for example, this clumsy sentence:

> Rogers (1967), however, took issue with Buber (1952) over the question of evil: with May (1956), Buber had challenged

Rogers's apparent failure to address what has been called 'the problem of evil' (Brown 1967, Davidson 1984).

A tidier and more easily read sentence might be:

Rogers was sometimes accused of ignoring the question of evil (Buber 1952, May 1956).

Remember, too, to pay attention to the way that you format references in your essay. In the next paragraphs, we consider the Harvard and Vancouver methods of referencing. Both are frequently used in academic essays and in journal papers. Again, it is essential to check with your lecturer about the style of referencing that you are to use.

The Harvard system of referencing

The Harvard system of referencing is the one in which the name of the author and the date of publication appear in the body of the text and the full reference is listed at the end. Here is an example of the end of a paper in which the system has been used:

The writer has discussed the question of whether or not all clients should attend group therapy sessions in another paper (Brown 1987). Other writers have also discussed this issue, most notably Davis (1989) and Anderson (1990, 1991).

References

Anderson, P. (1990) Group therapy for in patients. *British Journal of Group Work*, **2**(4), 34–46.

Anderson, P. (1991) *Working With Groups*. Heinemann, Oxford.

Brown, D. (1991) Does group work make a difference? *Nursing Times*, **3**(5), 67–68.

Davis, L. (1989) *Against Groups*. Pan, London.

The points that you need to pay close attention to with the Harvard system of referencing are:

- Only the author's surname and the date of publication appear in the body of the text.
- In the reference list at the end of the essay, references are listed alphabetically by author.

- If an author has two publications in the same year and both are referred to, one is called a and the other b (e.g. Brown 1989a, 1989b) Full references are listed at the end, noting, correctly, reference a and reference b.
- In the reference list, the following are always listed and in this order: author's surname, author's initials, date of publication, title, publisher, place of publication. This is true when the publication is a book. For journal references, the order is as follows: author's surname, author's initials, date of publication, title of journal, volume number, issue number, pages. In the list, book titles are underlined or italicised. With references to journal papers, the name of the journal is underlined or italicised. It is important to get this right.

Some variants of the basic Harvard system

The basic Harvard system, then, involves the quotation of a surname and date, in brackets, in the main body of the text, with a full list of the references used, alphabetically by author, at the end of the text. There is a range of variations of this method and some of these are now described. These should be used as guidelines: there are sometimes 'local' variations in colleges and departments: personal preferences of lecturers and journal editors sometimes mean that approaches other than the ones listed here are used. Overall, the really important issue is that you are consistent in the way that you use references.

Works having two or three authors

Where a book or paper has two or three authors, these should be listed, in the order they appear in the original publication, in brackets with the date, in the text, e.g. (Brown, Smith and Jones 2003).

Works having more than three authors

Where a book or paper has more than three authors, the first should be quoted, followed by '*et al.*' in brackets, before the date, e.g. (Davies *et al.* 2004). In the list of references, at the back of the paper, *all* authors should be quoted in full. Some authorities prefer the use of '*et al.*' for books and papers that have more than two authors while others prefer to use it where there are two or more.

When a work has a corporate author

When a book or paper has no individual's name offered as author, it is usual to quote the organisation's name as the author, e.g. (British

Association of Health Workers 1999). An alternative is to *abbreviate* the organisation when you cite the reference the first time and, subsequently, to use that abbreviation. Example:

> *First citation*: This point was developed in a report on handwashing in the workplace (British Association of Health Workers [BAHW] 1999).

> *Second and subsequent citations*: The issue of washing hands both before and after handling food has been dealt with elsewhere (BAHW 1999).

When an author has published more than one book or paper in the same year

It is sometimes necessary to quote various papers by the same author published in the same year. In this case, it is usual to designate each 'a', 'b', 'c' and so on, e.g. (James 2002a, 2002b, 2002c). In the reference list, these are written out in full, complete with the appropriate letter after the date.

When a reference is to a chapter in a book edited by another author

It is quite often necessary to quote a chapter (by one author) in a book edited by another. Here, the name of the author of the chapter is cited in brackets, with the date. In the reference list, full details of both the chapter and the book are written out. Here is an example of both the reference in the text and the listing in the reference list.

> Various writers have discussed the question of health-care funding in areas where there is a large population of elderly people. Davies (2004) has suggested that local funding is rarely adequate.

> Davies, P.D. (2004) Local funding of health care. In: P. Brown and T. Smith, *The Economics of Local Health Care*, Nelson Thornes, Cheltenham.

When one author is quoted by another

Sometimes, it is impossible to go back to primary sources and to find out directly what an author wrote. In this case, it becomes necessary to use another author's quoting of the original author. Imagine, for example, that you have picked up a book called *Counselling in the Health Services* by an author called David Smith, published in 2003. In this book, Smith writes as follows:

The concept of empathy is a difficult one. We probably all know what if feels like to be understood but being totally understood is another matter. Brown writes about it as follows:

> No single person can ever fully understand another. The idea that empathy is something that can be taught is fraught with problems. We do not get 'taught' to empathise. Instead, we learn it through the process of growing up with other people (Brown 2002).

If you wanted to use this information about Brown in your own work, you would have to quote it as follows:

> Brown (cited by Smith 2003) suggests that we probably cannot be *taught* to empathise but have to learn it through the process of living alongside others.

In the reference list, you would quote the Smith book as follows:

> Smith, D. (2003) *Counselling in the Health Services*, Butterworth-Heinemann, Oxford.

This is a rather complicated issue. Wherever possible, it is best to avoid this sort of citation. Wherever possible, go back to the original source of the information. In this case, you would try to find Brown's book and work directly from that. It is certainly not good practice to rely on one or two textbooks and to use lots of 'cited by' references by pulling out information from these one or two sources.

When two authors have the same surname

When two different authors, with the same name, are referred to in a paper of manuscript, it is important to include their *initials* so that the reader can be sure about to which one you are referring. For example:

> I.J. Davies (2003) discusses a range of issues to do with GP practice and the use of antibiotics. In another paper, P.D. Davies (2003) identifies some of the more common side effects of the broad-spectrum antibiotics.

Personal communications

Personal communications may include letters, memos, telephone conversations and face-to-face conversations. Generally, it is not good practice to cite personal communications in papers and manuscripts but sometimes this is the only way of identifying a source of information. When 'personal communication' is cited, the reference is only placed in the body of the text and is not included in the reference list at the end of the document. It is usual to offer the initials and surname of the other person, along with the full date. For example:

> For some, it is important to help depressed patients to externalise aggression by forcing the person into a heated debate or argument (J. Richards, personal communication, 12th May 2004).

It is important to learn the correct format for the Harvard referencing system. Once learned, it becomes second nature in the using. Also, many published books and journals use the system so you will quickly come to recognise its use. Until recently, it has been the most popular form of referencing system. The Vancouver system seems to be catching it up.

The Vancouver system of referencing

In the Vancouver system, a series of numbers is used to indicate that a reference is being used. Those references are then listed at the end of the paper, in numerical order as those numbers appeared in the text. The above example, written with the Vancouver system of referencing, would appear like this:

> The writer has discussed the question of whether or not all clients should attend group therapy sessions in another paper (1). Other writers have also discussed this issue, most notably Davis (2) and Anderson (3, 4).

References

1. Brown D. Does group work make a difference? *Nursing Times* 2003; **3**(5): 67–68.

2. Davis L. *Against Groups*. London: Pan, 2002.

3. Anderson P. Group therapy for in patients. *British Journal of Group Work* 2000; **2**(4): 34–46.

4. Anderson P. *Working With Groups*. Oxford: Heinemann, 2001.

The advantages of the Vancouver system are that it is easier on the eye when you are reading a paper. All you see is a series of numbers and, in printed text, these numbers are usually set as superscript (the number is set in a small type face above the line). Also, you can easily check the reference at the end of the paper by looking up the number. On the other hand, the Vancouver system does not always refer you to the name of the author. Also, it is very difficult to make adjustments to once you try to add references to a paper that you are writing. Each time you add a reference, you upset the numbering system. The Vancouver system of referencing is quite widely used in journals and books and you should seek advice from the journal you're writing in, for details of its idiosyncratic use.

Whatever type of referencing system you use, you must use it correctly and consistently. A common fault is to mix the styles and to quote author, date of publication and a number in the text. You should avoid this and learn both systems.

Examples of referencing styles to avoid

In reading other people's essays, it is possible to come across all sorts of 'hybrid' styles of referencing. The following are examples of methods of referencing to avoid. In each case, the writer has broken the fairly simple rules stipulated under the Harvard or Vancouver formats.

✋ *Over to you*

Identify what is wrong with each example in the box below:

Example 1
ANDREWS (2003) has written extensively about the use of computers in social work. He has suggested, as has JONES (2004) that all social workers should use portable computers for notetaking and record keeping.

Example 2
Andrews, J. (2003) has written extensively about the use of computers in social work. He has suggested, as has Jones, P.D. (2004) that all social workers should use portable computers for notetaking and record keeping.

Example 3
Andrews, Peter (2003) has written extensively about the use of computers in social work. He has suggested, as has Jones, Philip (2004) that all social workers should use portable computers for notetaking and record keeping.

Example 4
Andrews 2003 (1) has written extensively about the use of computers in social work. He has suggested, as has Jones 2004 (2) that all social workers should use portable computers for notetaking and record keeping.

Example 5
Andrews 2003 has written extensively about the use of computers in social work. He has suggested, as has **Jones 2004** that all social workers should use portable computers for notetaking and record keeping.

Diagrams and figures

In some health service courses, essays may require diagrams. There are two things to say about these:

- Only use them if they really do illuminate your text in a way that words could not
- Keep them simple. Avoid complicated drawings of circles and arrows. Some readers may assume that you are suggesting that there is some sort of mathematical or spatial relationship between the various elements of a complicated diagram.

Health-care literature went through a phase of writers including complicated, circular diagrams. Perhaps these had been borrowed from the business and educational literatures that also tended to favour them. As a rule, keep them simple or leave them out all together.

Tables are sometimes essential. If you are referring to numerical data in a research report, you are likely to need to show some of the numbers. Again, keep the tables simple. Avoid too many lines. Prefer horizontal lines to vertical ones and do not show too many numbers in one table.

Layout

How you present your essay is important. Figure 7.1 overleaf illustrates the points that you should consider when planning your essay manuscript. Features of this layout include:

- Wide margins of about 2–3 cm
- Double spacing
- Indented paragraphs after the first under each heading
- Bold or underlined subheadings.

Key points | **Top tips**

Gillett offers, amongst others, the following pointers about essay presentation:

1. The question should be accurately written out, at the top of the paper. This is important, not just for the assessor, but also so that in years to come you can clearly identify the subject you were writing about!

2. The date of the assignment and course details, with your name or candidate number should be clearly noted, together with the location of your study centre or institution, if appropriate.

3. The organisation of the material should be clear, with logical paragraph construction, appropriate use of headings, wide margins for the assessor to write in, etc.

4. Correct spelling and diligent proof-reading are important, as well as good use of English – clear, concise and jargon-free. If you know that your spelling is poor, ask a colleague or friend who can spell to help you. It would be unusual for marks to be deducted for spelling errors, but it can be very irritating to the assessor.

5. A clear original or a good photocopy should be presented, i.e. one that does not have grubby looking pages with words disappearing off the edge of the page.

6. Remember to number the pages.

7. Include an approximate word count.

8. *Always, always keep a copy of any work that you hand in.* It has been known for work to be lost *en route* to the assessor. Remember that one essay may be marked by two or three different people and so the potential for it being lost is quite high!

Gillett 1990, p. 93

⚷ Keywords

Plagiarism
The attempt at passing off someone else's written work as your own – in other words, copying straight out of books, articles and papers

Plagiarism

Avoid **plagiarism** like the plague: the name, alone, should put you off. It is not permitted in any sort of written work, although it crops up mostly in essays. To plagiarise is illegal and is one of the very few things that can get you thrown straight off a university or college course. Sometimes, it is done unwittingly. Some people take notes directly out of books and papers and then transfer them into essays. Others, I think, don't *know* that it is wrong to copy directly. Nor is plagiarism always clear-cut. In the following examples I show varieties of what is and what is not plagiarism, with a borderline case in between.

Sample text

The following is an (imaginary) piece of text from a book called *Counselling for Health Workers* by Allan Jones, published in 2004 by Jacobs & Jacobs, London.

There are debates about whether or not counselling 'works'. Various outcome studies have been conducted (e.g. Davies 2002, Andrews 2003, Jowett 2003) in which researchers have tested clients both before and after counselling sessions as an attempt to try to establish (or otherwise) the efficacy of counselling. The problem with undertaking these sorts of studies is that they cannot control all of the variables that

ASPECTS OF AIDS AND HIV

John Brown: June 2004

The number of people being diagnosed as being human immunodeficiency virus (HIV) positive or having acquired immune deficiency syndrome (AIDS) is increasing. There is growing evidence that HIV is spreading in the UK by various means in both heterosexual and homosexual populations (Donoghue *et al*. 1989, Pye *et al*. 1989, Brewer 2003). Two decades after the emergence of HIV and AIDS most nurses and health professionals will have personal or professional experience of knowing someone who is HIV-positive or who has AIDS (Connor and Kingman 1989, Miller 1990, Rondahl *et al*. 2003). Despite health-care professionals expressing empathetic attitudes towards HIV-infected patients and a low degree of fear of HIV infection, a significant (36%) number suggested that they would avoid caring for HIV-infected patients if at all possible (Rondahl *et al*. 2003).

The changing picture

While there are indications that people are beginning to listen to the call for safe sex, there is also evidence that people associate AIDS with being homosexual and that moral positions are still being held (Wellings and Wadsworth 1990, Fitzpatrick and Milligan 1990). While the notion of AIDS as punishment meted out by God is less popular now, it is still possible to find those who are ignorant about the condition and less than sympathetic to the people who have it (Gaze 1987, Frankenberg 1990). Wellings and Wadsworth (1990) reporting *British Social Attitudes* noted that 55% of their respondents agreed with the statement that 'AIDS sufferers have only themselves to blame'. It has been suggested that media attempts to change people's attitudes towards AIDS have been less than successful (Kitzinger 1990).It has also been suggested that AIDS has features in common with epidemics in Europe such as the Black Death of the 14th century (Last 1988). What is less clear is the degree to which such comparisons add to people's attitudes towards AIDS and AIDS related conditions. For, as Connor and Kingman (1989) point out:

> AIDS is not, in short, a highly contagious disease, so it is not strictly speaking a 'modern plague', equivalent to the Black Death which decimated Europe in the Middle Ages. (Connor and Kingman 1990: 3).

These differing viewpoints and perspectives indicate how perceptions of AIDS vary. Given that these opposing viewpoints are offered by experts in the field, it is reasonable to expect that such diversity of perception also exists amongst the general public and amongst nurses.

Figure 7.1 *Example of essay layout*

are present. Do clients get better because of counselling or do they 'just recover'? Do their families help them and support them while they are being counselled? What is it that 'works'? The counselling or the relationship that they have with the counsellor? All of these things (and, no doubt, many others) make outcome studies difficult.

Outright plagiarism

In the following example, a student has simply copied out the above text and included it, without any sort of reference, in her own essay. This is an obvious case of plagiarism and, if spotted by an examiner, would land the student in serious trouble.

> Research into counselling is difficult. There are debates about whether or not counselling 'works'. Various outcome studies have been conducted (e.g. Davies 2002, Andrews 2003, Jowett 2003) in which researchers have tested clients both before and after counselling sessions as an attempt to try to establish (or otherwise) the efficacy of counselling. The problem with undertaking these sorts of studies is that they cannot control all of the variables that are present. Do clients get better because of counselling or do they 'just recover'? Do their families help them and support them while they are being counselled? What is it that 'works'? The counselling or the relationship that they have with the counsellor? All of these things (and, no doubt, many others) make outcome studies difficult.

A borderline case

The following example shows that plagiarism is not always black and white. Some people quote direct chunks of other people's work and offer a reference to the original work. In the following example, though, it is still unclear what the student is claiming as her own work and what she is expecting the reader to attribute to Jones.

> Research into counselling is difficult. Jones (2004) points out that there are debates about whether or not counselling 'works'. Various outcome studies have been conducted (e.g. Davies 2002, Andrews 2003, Jowett 2003) in which researchers have tested clients both before and after counselling sessions as an attempt to try to establish (or otherwise) the efficacy of counselling. The problem with undertaking these sorts of studies is that they cannot control all of the variables that are present. This means that

attempts at really clarifying whether or not counselling makes a difference are likely to be thwarted.

In this example, the student has skilfully (or unskilfully, depending on your point of view) intermeshed Jones's direct words with her own. Some might argue that the inclusion of a reference to Jones's work renders the above example acceptable. The fact is, though, that the student is still passing off Jones's work as if it were her own.

Not plagiarism

The following two examples show how the student might have tackled the issue by using Jones's work but not attempting to claim the words as her own.

In the first example, the student paraphrases what Jones has written and makes it clear when she is referring, directly, to Jones's work. She does not quote directly from the work of Jones.

> Attempts at trying to find out whether or not counselling works have been problematic. Jones (2004) points out that outcome studies are likely to be difficult because so many variables are at work. Jones suggests that in outcome studies it is difficult to know whether or not it is the 'counselling' that works or if other factors, such as the client's relatives or even the relationship between client and counsellor contribute to the client getting better.

In the second example, the student quotes directly from Jones's work but makes it very clear that she is using a direct quote by indenting the paragraph and citing the reference and page number. This is not plagiarism but appropriate quotation from another writer's work.

> It is nearly always difficult to find out whether or not counselling makes a difference to clients. Jones (2004) writes clearly and at length on this topic. He argues that:

> > Various outcome studies have been conducted (e.g. Davies 2002, Andrews 2003, Jowett 2003) in which researchers have tested clients both before and after counselling sessions as an attempt to try to establish (or otherwise) the efficacy of counselling. The problem with undertaking these sorts of studies is that they cannot control all of the variables that are present (Jones 2004, p. 24).

It is almost impossible to overstate how important it is to guard against plagiarism. In recent years there have been court cases over students who have had their degrees withdrawn after it has been established that their essays and/or dissertations contained large chunks of other people's work. If you have any doubts about whether or not you are plagiarising as you write, check your work with a colleague or a lecturer.

Checking your essay

Before you hand it in, it is essential that you read through and check your essay thoroughly. One of the drawbacks of using a word-processing program is that it allows you to work *too* quickly and easily, once you have learned the program. It checks your spelling (but does not pick up differences between words such as 'there' and 'their'), it allows you to review your work on the screen, before you print it out. And this may not be the best way of doing things. In my experience, it is always wise to print out a 'hard' copy of your essay and to sit down, with a pen, and work through it for spelling, punctuation, style and content. What looked right on the computer screen may not look so good when it is printed out. It may, of course, look much better.

Key points **Top tips**

Giles and Hedge (1994) offer a useful checklist of points for checking an essay, project or assignment:

1. Have you kept your audience in mind throughout your essay?
2. Have you said what you meant to say? Does your writing convey your intended message?
3. Have you been consistent and followed the conscientious of the genre in which you are writing?
4. Have you signalled the organisation of your text in the most appropriate way?
5. Have you given your writing to anyone else to read in order to make sure they understand it?
6. Are your arguments logical?
7. Have you 'hedged your bets' when necessary?
8. Have you used enough evaluation? Is your evaluation careful and precise?
9. If you know you have trouble with some grammatical points, have you checked these?
10. Has every sentence got a subject and a verb?
11. Do your verbs agree with your subjects?
12. Do your sentences have agreement of tense, number and person?
13. Have you checked your spelling? If you have used a word-processing spelling checker, have you then checked the spelling yourself?
14. Have you checked your punctuation?

Giles and Hedge 1994

Binding

Unless you are given specific instructions about a particular form of binding for your essay, it is probably better not to bind it at all. Binders of any sort add weight to a pile of essays and the examiner has to carry them, send them to the external examiner and have them posted back. All this can turn out to be very heavy and expensive if each essay is separately bound. If you must use a binder, use a very simple, transparent one. Don't use ring binders or lever arch files. Nor be tempted to file each page of your essay in a separate, plastic cover within a binder. This makes it almost impossible for the marker to write notes on your essay directly.

The best approach is probably to have a title page on the front of your essay (see Figure 7.2 for an example) and simply to staple the top left-hand corner of your essay. This, in the end, makes for much easier 'handling' of your essay and will usually be much appreciated by the person who has to mark it.

Whatever you do, don't cut out an illustration from a magazine and stick it on the title page to illustrate your essay.

If in any doubt about any of these issues, check with the person to whom you will be handing the essay. Remember, though, what

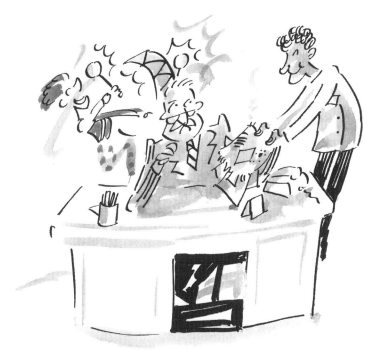

Your work should be submitted in a simple and appropriate way. The content is more important than a fancy presentation.

University of Blackheath
Department of Occupational Therapy
MSc in Health Care Studies

A review of the literature on the history of occupational therapy
Jane Hamersmith

Submitted on 22nd December 2003
2496 words

Figure 7.2 *Example of an essay cover page*

counts is the *content* of your essay and not your ability to present it in an unusual and arresting way.

Feedback

Unfortunately, there are few standards when it comes to the marking of essays. Nor is there consistency about how much or how little written feedback any given tutor or lecturer will give you about your essay. Clearly, notes at the bottom of your essay such as 'good' or 'well written' are of little help. The more conscientious marker will go through your essay and offer you some commentary on it. Sometimes, this will be in the form of numbered annotations running through the work. In other words, the marker puts a '1' or a '2' in the margin of your work and on a separate sheet offers you notes about the '1' and the '2'. In this way, she can almost engage in a dialogue with you about your work.

Other markers and other colleges award marks for your work according to a grid of some sort. Here, you will be allocated a certain percentage of marks for a particular aspect of your essay. There may, for example, be marks awarded in a similar format to the following:

Use of research	25%
Use of other literature	25%
Appropriate referencing	15%
Critical debate of the issues	25%
Layout and presentation	10%

Whatever method is used, you need to know exactly where you stand in relation to your work. If you feel that the written comments on your essay are not sufficient to allow you to learn from them, make sure that you make an appointment to see the marker and discuss your work. Remember, too, that in many colleges and universities, the initial marking is provisional. Most college work is moderated by an external examiner, who always has the last word about marks awarded. Make sure you know whether or not your work has been or will be seen and moderated by an external examiner. Some colleges and universities also have a system by which you can be asked to attend a viva or oral examination of all or part of your work. This is usually done if your work falls along a borderline – between degree classifications, between 'pass' and 'fail' or between 'pass' and 'distinction'.

In conclusion, all the issues relating to writing that have been discussed so far apply to writing essays. Keep sentences and paragraphs short. Write to express your ideas, not to impress. Don't try to be clever but express your ideas clearly. The sociologist C. Wright Mills summed it up when he wrote:

> To overcome the academic *prose* you have first to overcome the academic *pose*.
>
> Wright Mills 1959

RRRRRRapid recap

Check your progress so far by working through each of the following questions.

1. What does 'brainstorming' mean?
2. List three ways of collecting information for an essay.
3. What is meant by the term 'plagiarism'?

If you have difficulty with more than one of the questions, read through the section again to refresh your understanding before moving on.

References

Giles, K. and Hedge, N. (1994) *The Manager's Good Study Guide*. Open University Press, Milton Keynes.

Gillett, H. (1990) *Study Skills: a guide for health care professionals*. Distance Learning Centre, South Bank Polytechnic, London.

Wright Mills, C. (1959) *The Sociological Imagination*. Penguin, Oxford.

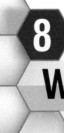

8

Writing theses and dissertations

Research? Anyone can do that.

Student, to the author

Learning outcomes

By the end of this chapter you should be able to:

- Understand the difference between a thesis and a dissertation
- Plan a research proposal
- Review the literature for your research and write a literature review
- Know when (and when not) to use footnotes.

Dissertation or thesis?

Labels can complicate matters. Just so we are clear what we are talking about, for the purposes of this chapter a dissertation is what an undergraduate writes in her final year and what a masters student writes as part of the requirements for her degree. The masters dissertation is usually a research report but it is also possible, in some colleges, to complete a literature-based dissertation. In essence, this is an extended review of the literature, although some colleges also ask for the inclusion of a research proposal as part of the dissertation. A thesis is what a doctoral student hands in as the final report of her research.

Following an oral examination (or viva) the doctoral student is awarded a PhD on the strength of the thesis and her performance at the oral.

In the USA and Canada, the labels are reversed. Masters students do theses and PhD students do dissertations.

An undergraduate dissertation in the UK is usually about 10,000 words in length. A taught masters degree dissertation is usually about 20,000. MPhil dissertations are usually up to about 60,000 words and a PhD thesis can be up to about 100,000 words. In practice, few examiners really want to read a double-volume, 100,000 word pair of tomes. If possible, it is usually better to write to under the upper limit. Some examiners refuse to mark works that are over the word limit. Others have some sort of penalty system for students who write too much. Why make life more difficult? After discussion with your tutor, it is likely that these maxima are useful ones to work to:

Bachelors dissertation:	8500 words
Taught masters dissertation:	18,000 words
MPhil dissertation:	50,000 words
PhD thesis:	60–70,000 words.

As far as is reasonably possible, avoid running to two volumes.

Content

As we have seen, a dissertation or thesis is usually also a research report. As such, the report will strongly echo a research proposal. Most such reports will contain the following chapters:

- **Abstract** – A short statement of less than 200 words summarising what your dissertation or thesis is about. Use these words carefully. The abstract is all that many people will read of your work. It will appear in abstracting journals and on research databases if it is submitted for a masters degree or PhD. Write the abstract after you have completed your work.

- **Acknowledgements** – Record your thanks to your supervisor and to your family. Go easy. I read an acknowledgement recently to the family dog. This is taking things a little far.

- **Introduction** – This is a short chapter that offers an overview of what is to come

- **Chapter 1** – Literature review
- **Chapter 2** – Aims of the study
- **Chapter 3** – Methodology
- **Chapter 4** – Analysis
- **Chapter 5** – Findings
- **Chapter 6** – Discussion of findings
- **Chapter 7** – Conclusions
- **Chapter 8** – Applications and limitations
- **References**
- **Appendices.**

It is not usual to index your dissertation or thesis, although I always think that this would be extremely useful. I hope that it becomes a standard feature as more and more people work with word-processing programs. There is rarely any need to go beyond 10 chapters. If you do write more than 10, you are likely to be writing rather superficially. Avoid too many appendices: they can appear to be page-filling and often are. Also avoid a bibliography unless your tutor has asked for one. The difference between a reference list and a bibliography is this. A reference list is a listing of all of the works that you have referred to directly in your dissertation or thesis. A bibliography is a separate listing of other books that are related to the topic but are not referred to in your work. In practice, bibliographies are very easy to compile, especially with the use of CD-ROM and other searching facilities. Bibliographies that are compiled in this way are merely a list of books and articles that the researcher has managed to find on the particular topic. Generally, it is better to stick to a reference list only.

Key points | **Top tips**

- Be methodical. Keep detailed notes about your work and always back up your computer files
- Make sure that the bibliographical references you collect are complete in every detail and that you know how to find the books and papers in question.

What should go in the appendices? There is often debate in academic departments about what should go in and what should be left out of the appendices of dissertations and theses (or even whether or not there should be appendices at all). Sommer and Sommer offer the following list of things that might be included in the appendices of a technical report:

- Score sheets, questionnaires or observation sheets used in the study. An exception would be instruments that are commonly used and widely available. These can be omitted.
- Detailed tables and charts primarily for reference purposes. Tables and figures necessary for the reader's understanding should be placed in the results section.
- List of technical terms. For a general audience, technical terms should also be defined as they occur in the text.
- Other relevant documents not essential to the reader's comprehension of the report. These might include the sign-up sheet for recruiting subjects, interviewer instructions, instructions for coding interview data, the follow-up letter to respondents who did not reply, etc. (Sommer and Sommer 1991).

In the appendices of qualitative studies, it is not unusual to include examples of interview transcripts and examples of the coding of those transcripts.

Planning your research project

The first thing you will be asked to do when you begin to plan your research is to write a research proposal. It is worth taking some time over this. It is important to bear in mind that your research must be achievable. Most people tend to overestimate what they can do in the time that they have. This is as true of PhD candidates as it is of undergraduates.

The research proposal

These are the headings that you can use for a research proposal. Check with your supervisor that they are the ones that she would like you to use.

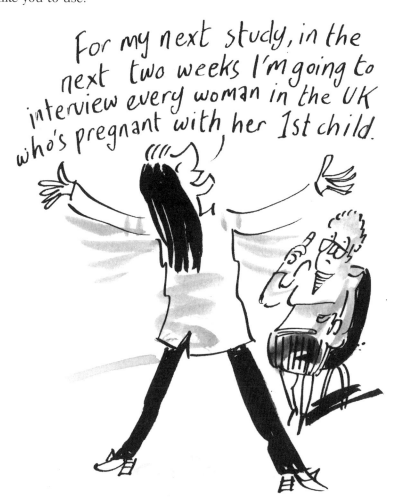

Make sure your plans are achievable.

- **Title** – Keep this short and descriptive. Avoid 'journalistic' tiles such as *The Baby and the Bathwater? Health-Care Cuts in the Provision of Community Care*. Instead, consider a straightforward title that tells the reader precisely what your study is about, e.g. *A Descriptive Study of the Economics of Community Care in a Rural Setting*.

- **Rationale** – Why do you want to do this research? How does it fit in with what has gone before? This should be about two paragraphs in length and place your research in context.

- **Aims** – Write about three research aims. Only use a hypothesis if you are using an experimental design. Only use an experimental design if you really know what you are doing. Take advice.

- **Sample** – How will you select out respondents from a total population? In the social sciences, it is rare to be able to contact a random sample. In a descriptive, qualitative study, numbers are not so important as the quality of the responses. Be clear about the sampling procedures for both qualitative and quantitative methodologies.

- **Method** – Here you should describe what it is you are going to do. Are you going to do some interviews? Are you going to use a questionnaire? If so, are you going to devise your own questionnaire or will you use someone else's? How will you check for the validity and reliability of your instrument? All of these details should be included in this section of your proposal.

- **Ethical considerations** – Will you have to go before an ethics committee? If so, what preparations have you made? Usually, if you are going to include patients or clients in your sample, you will be required to send your proposal to a local ethics committee. Do make sure that you are clear about your responsibilities in this field.

- **Financial considerations** – How will you pay for the various aspects of your research? Do not forget that you may have a large postage bill if you send out questionnaires. You will also have to pay for paper and for binding the final report. Do not assume that your college will pay for these things.

- **A short CV** – Write a two-page curriculum vitae in which you describe your own background in terms of education, jobs, publications and so forth. The aim of the CV in this case is to support your proposal and to show that you have the relevant experience to complete the research that you have in mind.

- **Timetable** – Write out a plan of action. The 'rule of thirds' is sometimes useful here. One third of your research time should be devoted to searching the literature. Another third will be taken up with data collection and analysis. The final third will see you writing your dissertation or thesis. On the other hand, it is also good practice to write up your work as you go.

Writing a research proposal is an important aspect of writing. Take time preparing it and then spend a little time or money in having it laser printed. Keep a copy for yourself and submit at least two copies to your supervisor.

Key points Top tips

- Make your dissertation or thesis interesting! Just because it is an academic work does not mean that it has to be dull
- Check everything: dates, facts, references, spelling, grammar, layout, binding, word limit
- Keep an eye on deadlines for submission of work.

Supervision

All research projects for degrees and higher degrees are supervised. The supervisor may be allocated to you or you may choose one. Make sure that you both get on together and that the supervisor has the right background to supervise your work.

You should be able to expect certain things from a supervisor. Here is a checklist of things to ask for:

- Clear guidance on how to proceed with a particular part of your study
- Regular feedback on any written work that you hand in
- Help with methodology and analysis
- Guidance on how to write up your project
- Support and interest
- Regular meetings.

For your part, you should be prepared to work for your supervisor. The supervisor will not be doing the research for you. She should be able to expect the following from you:

- Regular written reports
- Motivation
- Ability to work independently
- Awareness of how to use the method that you have chosen
- Realistic aims that you negotiate together.

Be prepared to compromise. As with most relationships, there needs to be give and take. It is easy to get carried away in research and think that there is only one way to do things. Your supervisor may have other ideas. Listen to her carefully, particularly if she has direct experience of the methodology you are using. Also, do not expect your supervisor to do everything for you. It is your responsibility to read up on methods and analysis. It is also your responsibility to be aware of and familiar with the literature in your particular field. It is unrealistic to expect your supervisor to know all about the literature in the area of your study.

Reviewing the literature

One of the first elements in the research process is a review of the literature. The literature review is used to demonstrate a number of things. It can:

- Demonstrate your knowledge of the writing and research in your chosen field
- Put your research into context – it can show how your project will contribute (even if only to a small degree) to the available knowledge in the field
- Help you to understand what other researchers have done
- Alert you to particular methodological problems
- Give you a greater understanding of the research process.

First, become aware of how to use bibliographies and abstracting journals in your library. These books list all the recent publications of work within your particular field of study. Also, get to know how to use the CD-ROM. CD-ROM offers you a very quick entry to huge numbers of bibliographical references. Learn how to trim down the numbers generated by the computer to a more manageable size.

Next, make sure that you record every reference that you think may be of use. If you use CD-ROM you can print out the details or you can download them to disk. Then, make decisions about which journal papers or books you will need to order through your library. Before you put in orders, check that the library does not already stock the papers or books that you need. Interlibrary loans cost a lot of money. Many academic libraries carry back issues of journals and books that are not displayed. Ask the librarian to show you the 'stacks'.

As you collect offprints of papers and collect books, begin to make detailed notes. Note, particularly, whether a given paper is of one of these sorts:

- **An opinion piece** – these may be editorials or single pages in weekly magazines or journals. Clearly, they only represent one person's opinion and cannot be held to be as 'weighty' as other sorts of publication. Do not use them on their own to support an argument.

- **A theory paper** – these are logically argued and properly referenced papers that present you with a theoretical position or that review the literature. Every so often an academic or researcher will actually publish a review of the literature. These are particularly useful if you are just starting out in a field of study. They are useful, too, as role models for the writing of your own literature review.

- **Research reports** – these are probably the most useful sorts of paper. They tell you what research has already been done. The tell you about the sample, method and analysis of findings. They present and discuss the findings and also lead you to the literature.

On your reference cards or in your computer database, make notes of which sort of paper you are dealing with. Then, make notes of what is in a particular paper. If you are likely to want to use direct quotations from the paper (and always use these sparingly), make a careful copy of the quotation and write down the page number next to it. Always offer page numbers when you make reference to direct quotations in your report.

Key points **Top tips**

Gash (1989) offers particular reasons why you should work more often with journal articles than with books when carrying out a search of the literature. She suggests that the significant characteristics of this type of publication are as follows.

- Journals contain the most recent material on the subject. This is because journal issues are published far more quickly and frequently than books.

- Journals are able to publish papers that are too short, too ephemeral, too controversial or too obscure to warrant publication in book form. The commercial success of a journal does not depend on the demand for one paper in one issue. A book must sell on its own merits.

- Collectively, journal literature will give an overview of the current state of a subject. Retrospectively, it will enable past trends to be identified and followed (Gash 1989, p. 11).

Writing up

When you write up your research review, try to avoid the rather dull listing of everything you have read. The aim of a literature review is not only to identify what you have read but for you to offer a critical review of what you have read. Therefore, you should become aware of shortcomings of method or analysis in a research report. You should also be aware of faulty argument or logic in theory papers. You should never just list what you have read, as in the extract in Figure 8.1. Instead, comment on the findings that you report. Offer a critique of the sampling, methodology and findings that the researcher offers. Indicate in what ways those researchers' findings fit in with your study.

> Brown (2001) found that 60% of college students under the age of 21 had dental caries. Davis (2002, 2003) also carried out research that supported this finding. White (2004) suggested that college students do not brush their teeth as often as they should, while Andrews (2001) reported that most young people do not change their toothbrush frequently.

Figure 8.1 *Example of how not to write a literature review.*

A *critical* review might read something like the passage in Figure 8.2.

> Brown (2001) in a study of 200 college students in a North American college found that 60% of his sample had dental caries. It is important to note, though, that Brown used a convenience sample and this may have affected the outcome of his study. In other studies, Davies (2002, 2003) replicated Brown's study with much larger and randomly selected samples. While Davies found that large numbers of students had dental caries, he found that, in government surveys, *most* young people between the ages of 12 and 21 were reported to have at least one area of caries. Davies noted, too, a far wider range of possible causes for caries in the under-21-year-old age group than did Brown. Following Davies's recommendation that researchers should be cautious in drawing conclusions from small-scale dental studies, I am limiting my study to a review of the research literature on dental work between 2003 and the present.

Figure 8.2 *Example of how a critical review might be written.*

If you keep your reference cards or database system up to date, you will be able to sort your references into an order. Thus, you will find that you can organise your literature review under a series of headings and subheadings. Here, for example, is an extract of the ordering of a literature review about counselling:

1. **Definitions of counselling**
   Client-centred counselling
   Prescriptive counselling
   Other types of counselling
2. **Humanistic psychology**
   History
   Carl Rogers
   Humanistic principles
   Objections
3. **Counselling skills**
   Client-centred skills
   Six category intervention analysis
   Questioning
   Reflection
   Empathy building
   Checking for understanding
4. **Counselling and the health professions**
   Counselling in medicine
   Counselling in nursing
   Counselling in occupational therapy
   AIDS counselling
   Genetic counselling
   RELATE (marriage guidance).

What a literature review looks like

Many people, when they start working on writing up a dissertation or thesis, worry about how to start because they are unsure what a literature review 'looks' like. It is often possible to have a look at other people's dissertations or theses in the local college or university library. In the end, though, a variety of different styles can be used. Figure 8.3, by way of an example, offers the beginning of an imaginary literature review on a dissertation that is about group work in the health-care professions.

This is, of course, not the only way to write up the literature. As you read it through, you may have your own thoughts about the style and the use of references. Some might question the use of the 'overview' in the introduction or even the use of subheadings. However you do it, you have to find a way of 'laying out' what has been done before: both in the literature and through research. Also,

Introduction

In the past 20 years, much has been written about the importance of clear communication in the health-care professions (see, for example, Brown 1978, 1980, Davies 1980, 1981, Smith 1985, Walker 1990). The group format is an economical one in terms of both time and resources (Walker 1992). In the small group, a number of people can communicate quickly with others. The group format can be used for communication in educational settings (Anthony 1993), therapy contexts (Evelyn 1999, Arthur 1999) and as support systems (Brown 2000, Davies 2000).

In this first section, the following issues are discussed: the structure of small groups, group facilitation and the process of assessing the value of group work. In the second section, a review of the research into group work is offered along with a critical review of the use of groups in health-care settings.

The structure of small groups

For the purposes of discussion, therapy, support and learning, the 'small group' is often described as being composed of fewer than 20 participants (Andrews 1998, Smithers 2000, Webb 2000). As Webb (2000) pointed out, the advantages of such small numbers are clear: each person can have his or her say, issues and problems can be shared, the group can be reasonably easily managed and group members develop a sense of group identity. Others have also argued that there is a range of psychological advantages to encouraging people to communicate and work in groups (see, for example, Hampton 1996, Anderson and James 2001, 2002) and these will be discussed in some detail later in this review.

On the other hand, the small group can be problematic. For those who do not 'belong' to the group, the small group can appear claustrophobic (Webster 2001). While Webster was referring, in particular, to group therapy, his comments were supported by Davis (2002) who, in a study of 240 student occupational therapists, found that the quieter members of the group often wished that they could leave it and join in a more 'anonymous' lecture. Andrews (1997), reviewing a number of studies into group participation, also reported that when one or two members were of a very different age to the majority of group members, they often felt left out. Again, the issues of inclusion and group identity will be discussed in greater detail below.

In health-care settings, there have been various reports of work in small groups of under 20. Jones (2000) reported that small-group work can be useful in helping to support junior doctors working in stressful environments. Andrews (1995) described the use of small groups for helping people with mental health problems in community settings while Jackson (2001) discussed the use of small therapy groups in inpatient mental health settings. Jenks and Henderson (1996) argued for more research into the effectiveness of such groups and it is notable that what all the preceding papers have in common is that they were case studies of group work. None of them referred directly to research into groups or group work.

Figure 8.3 *Example of a part of a literature review*

that review should not merely be a 'list' of what has already been written, it should also offer critical commentary.

There is probably no such thing as the ideal literature review. While the better ones will be exhaustive in their coverage of what has gone before, no two are likely to be the same. If they were, we could simply record 'standard' reviews of various topics on to floppy disks, give away the copyright on them and encourage students to load the 'standard' review into the front of their dissertations or theses. The point of a literature review is also to illustrate how the student has thought about a particular field, how she does or does not understand the context of her study and to demonstrate the ability to summarise previous literature.

> **Key points** Top tips
>
> All the issues discussed in previous chapters about how to write apply to the writing of a literature review. Remember:
> - Write short sentences
> - Write short paragraphs
> - Use simple words
> - Define what you mean, as you go
> - Be critical of what you read and write
> - Aim to communicate and not to impress.

Again, all the things that apply to writing a literature review apply to writing the other chapters of your research report. If you use the layout suggested in Figure 8.3 for your report, you are likely to find that it is quite easy to head towards the word limit imposed on you. You will have to be selective about what you include and what you leave out.

At all times, bear in mind that your research report should not only convey your findings but should lay out your methodology so clearly that another researcher could work through your report and repeat the process that you worked through. It should be that clear. Also, you should at all times be aware of the weaknesses of your study. For examples of clear, easy-to-read and easy-to-replicate (at least in theory) studies, look at some of the psychological studies that were carried out 20 or 30 years ago. Consider, for example, Sidney Jourard's (1971) reports of his studies into self-disclosure. Some years ago, a colleague and I replicated some of Jourard's work and found it quite easy to work through his writing and replicate what he did almost exactly (Burnard and Morrison 1992). You should aim at this sort of clarity.

A particular use of footnotes

In previous chapters, I have suggested that, as a rule, it is not a good idea to use footnotes. They are distracting to the reader and have generally fallen into disuse. However, there are times, in the reporting of a qualitative study, when they can be useful. Qualitative methods have been widely described in the literature (see, for example, Glaser and Strauss 1967, Ashworth *et al.* 1986, Field and Morse 1985, Bryman 1988, Burnard and Morrison 1992). It has been suggested that qualitative methods describe *what sorts* of thing there are in the world, while quantitative methods describe *how many*.

Qualitative research reports individuals' perceptions, their subjective experiences and opinions.

Footnotes can be useful as a means of offering commentary on a piece of transcript of an interview. Most top-level word-processing programs can easily generate footnotes and will take care of their management. If, for instance, you remove a particular footnote, the rest will automatically be renumbered.

Commentary can be at the level of a discussion of certain aspects of the interview or it can involve an elaboration of what has been said by a particular respondent in the study. Such annotated interview transcripts can be used, in an appendix in the dissertation or thesis, to illustrate an example of one interview. Alternatively, such transcripts can be used as part of the reporting of findings, in the main body of the text. Figure 8.4 offers an example of the use of footnotes in annotating a research transcript.

Style of a research report

Writing a dissertation or a thesis is different to writing a book, article or paper. Polit and Hungler (1991) offer useful advice about the style of a research report:

> A scientific report is not an essay but rather a factual account of how and why a problem was studied and what results were obtained. The report should generally not include overtly subjective statements, emotionally laden statements or exaggerations. When opinions are stated, they should be clearly identified as such, with proper attribution if the opinion was expressed by another writer. In keeping with the goal of objective reporting, personal pronouns such as 'I' and 'my' and 'we' are often avoided, because the passive voice and impersonal pronouns do a better job of conveying impartiality. However, some journals are beginning to break with this tradition and are encouraging a greater balance between active and passive voice and first-person and third-person narration. If a direct presentation can be made without sacrificing objectivity, the result is usually more readable and lively.
>
> Polit and Hungler 1991

It was noted, earlier, that the rule against the 'first person' in journals is, quite quickly, being revised. It is also not uncommon for qualitative research reports to be written – at least in part – in the first person, with the researcher reporting his or her findings directly.

Researcher: Could you tell me a little about the training that you had as a counsellor?

Respondent: I trained for three years as a client-centred counsellor[1] – that was about five years ago. Then I did a short gestalt therapy[2] course. I suppose that I mostly use a humanistic approach[3] that is basically client-centred. I don't believe in the psycho-analytical approach.[4] I'm not sure that it's necessarily a good thing to always harp on the past like that. I know it suits some people but I . . . anyway, I would have to have further training in that sort of thing if I was to use that approach.[5]

Researcher: What do you *do* as a counsellor?

Respondent: That's a big question! Well, I do lots of things. I mean, first and foremost, I *listen*[6] to the client.[7] I think that listening is all-important, really. You can *say* all sorts of things but the important thing is that the client feels listened to. What else? Well, I use 'reflection'[8] a lot. I sort of echo back to the client what he or she has said. I think it can sound a bit daft if it's not used well. You know – the client is likely to say 'That's what I just said!' if you use it too much. In the end, though, I think it helps to keep the client 'on track'. It helps them to continue talking about a particular thing. That's important if you want to go deeper . . ..

Researcher: What does it mean to 'go deeper?'

1 An approach to counselling developed by Carl Rogers (1952, 1967, 1983). He first called it 'non-directive' counselling and later 'client-centred'. Generally, the aim is not to offer advice or to 'interpret' what the other person says but to help the other person to make his or her own life-decisions.

2 Gestalt therapy, a particular type of humanistic therapy developed by Fritz Perls. Sometimes described as an existential philosophy, it puts consider-able emphasis on the 'client' making his or her own decisions based on developing self-awareness through noticing small and large physiological, psy-chological and perceptual changes.

3 'Humanistic psychology', often described as the 'third force' in psychology, to distinguish it from psychodynamic psychology and behavioural psy-chology. It focuses particularly on subjective human experience. Carl Rogers, founder of the client-centred approach to counselling, was a key figure in the humanistic psychology movement. The movement is thought to have been named by Abraham Maslow, the American psychologist probably best known, latterly, for his 'hierarchy of needs'.

4 The psychoanalytical approach: part of a wider, psychological approach known as the psychodynamic school of psychology. The term 'psycho-analytical' usually refers to the work of Freud, whereas the term 'analytical' refers to that of Jung. The various approaches usually moot the existence of an 'unconscious' mind that is not readily accessible to the individual but may be accessed through various forms of therapy – most notably through psychoanalysis itself. It is notable that the respondent 'does not believe in it'.

5 Training as a psychoanalytical therapist usually involves entering a 'training analysis' – the therapist must first be analysed. It is questionable whether or not the respondent would remain a *counsellor* if she undertook this training. It seems more likely that she would then be operating as a *therapist*. This raises interesting questions about the differences between counselling and psychotherapy – issues taken up later in the interview. For a critique of both client-centred and psychodynamic therapies, see Mason (1989), who argued that all therapies involve the imposition of the therapist's values on the client.

6 The idea of listening being a central feature of counselling is emphasised in much of the counselling literature (see, for example, Rogers 1967, Heron 1983, Burnard 1990).

7 Note the use of the term *client* to describe the person who receives counselling. The term was probably first used by Carl Rogers in place of the term *patient*. It is widely used in counselling circles and, to a lesser degree, in psychotherapy.

8 A device, technique or skill widely used in counselling. It involves repeating back the last few words that the other person has spoken to 'jog' them to say more. Also widely used in television interviews. The respondent alludes to how 'artificial' it can seem if overused.

Figure 8.4 *Example of the use of footnotes in the annotation of an interview transcript in qualitative research*

Evaluation

What makes a good dissertation or thesis? The point has been debated frequently in universities and colleges and in the literature. Hansen and Waterman (1966) and Howard and Sharp (1983) offer the following criteria for judging your own and other's research:

- Evidence of an original investigation or the testing of ideas
- Competence in independent work or experimentation
- An understanding of appropriate techniques
- Ability to make critical use of published work and source materials
- Appreciation of the relationship of the special theme to the wider field of knowledge
- Worthy, in part, of publication
- Originality as shown by the topic researched or the methodology employed
- Distinct contribution to knowledge.

Not all these criteria will need to be applied to all dissertations and theses. There should, for example, be a considerable difference between an undergraduate final-year dissertation and a PhD thesis. The point, of course, is that there are no laid-down guidelines for exactly what this difference should be. Most people, when asked about this question (and I have asked a lot of people about it), talk about issues such as 'depth' and 'detail'. In my experience, few academics or others can state clearly what the differences are between different levels of research. This being the case, work through the above criteria and apply them to your own research.

Layout

As with essays, books and anything else you write, how you lay out your thesis or dissertation is important. Figure 8.5 illustrates the usual format for layout. Note the following features:

- Wide margins
- Double spacing
- Clear subheadings
- Indented paragraphs after the first under each heading or subheading or 'double-double' spacing between paragraphs.

Publishing

The final stage of the research process is the publication of the findings. This is an important element of research: the publication makes your findings available to other researchers just as you depended on others when you began your literature search. There are a number of ways of publishing your findings. Here are some of them:

CHAPTER 3

STAGE ONE: QUALITATIVE STUDY OF PERCEPTIONS

This chapter describes the first part of the data collection and analyses. It explores the following issues:

- The sample
- Ethical issues
- Access to the sample
- The interview method
- Methods of analysis of the interviews.

Introduction

The chapter describes the first stage of the study in which interviews were carried out to explore a small group of nurse tutors' and student nurses' perceptions of experiential learning.

Sample

It was decided to interview a group of 12 nurse tutors regarding their views of experiential learning. The criterion for inclusion in this group was that the nurse educator claimed to be using experiential learning methods in his/her work with student nurses. Following Bogdan and Taylor's (1982) suggestion about obtaining respondents, the researcher often asked the person who was being interviewed to recommend another person whom that respondent knew to be using experiential learning methods. This has also been called the snowballing approach to selecting a sample (Field and Morse 1985).

The snowballing approach was felt to be the best way to gain access to respondents who might talk authoritatively on the topic in hand. It was in line with the researcher's intention to explore the perceptions of people who were using or subject to experiential learning methods.

Figure 8.5 *Example of a dissertation layout*

- **As a 'short report'** – A number of journals publish a brief report of recently completed research. Sometimes there is payment for such reports. This is unlikely to be the case in the heavyweight journals.

- **As a journal paper** – Here, you submit your work to an academic journal. As we note in Chapter 9, it is usual practice for such journals to have submissions reviewed 'blind'. That is to say that the editor sends your manuscript to two reviewers, without disclosing your name. She then takes guidance from them as to whether or not your work should be published. You may be asked to rewrite part or all of your paper before it is published. If asked, do so.

- **As a series of papers** – In this case, you publish your methodology, your findings and various discussion papers as separate entities.

- **As a monograph** – There are a number of imprints of larger publishing houses (e.g. Avebury) who print hard backed monographs from camera-ready copy supplied by the researcher. Such companies may not offer you royalties but will guarantee speedy publication of your work. Again, such imprints usually seek advice on the quality of your work.

- **As a standard, commercial book** – In this case, you are likely to be asked to rewrite some or all of your research report to make it publishable. Be prepared to do this and read the chapter on writing books. Few, if any, publishers are likely to publish an entire dissertation or thesis, with the exception of the monograph series described above.

Do get your work published. You will enjoy seeing your work in print and so will other people. You are adding to the body of knowledge only if other people have access to your work. Also, having publications on your CV will make a difference to your career prospects, particularly if you intend teaching in a college or university, or if you want to do more research.

ЯЯЯЯЯ*Rapid recap*

Check your progress so far by working through each of the following questions.

1. What is the difference between a dissertation and a thesis?
2. What is the difference between a reference list and a bibliography?
3. What support can you expect from your dissertation/thesis supervisor?
4. What can your supervisor expect from you?

If you have difficulty with more than one of the questions, read through the section again to refresh your understanding before moving on.

References

Burnard, P. and Morrison, P. (1992) *Self Disclosure: A contemporary analysis*. Avebury, Aldershot.

Gash, S. (1989) *Effective Literature Searching for Students*. Gower, Aldershot.

Hansen, K.J. and Waterman, R.C. (1966) Evaluation of research in business education. *National Business Education Quarterly*, **35**, 81–84.

Howard, K. and Sharp, J.A. (1983) *The Management of a Student Research Project*. Gower, Aldershot.

Jourard, S. (1971) *Self-disclosure: An experimental analysis of the transparent self*. Wiley, New York.

Polit, D.F. and Hungler, B.P. (1991) *Nursing Research: Principles and methods,* 4th edn. J.B. Lippincott, Philadelphia, PA.

9

Writing articles

Learning outcomes

By the end of this chapter you should be able to:

- Understand the process and requirements for writing for magazines
- Understand the process and requirements for writing for journals.

I don't want to take up literature in a money-making spirit, or be very anxious about making large profits, but selling it at a loss is another thing altogether, and an amusement I cannot well afford.

Lewis Carroll to his publisher

It has been said before, but the best way to learn about something is to write about it. Once you have finished formal courses of teaching and learning, there is often a bit of a gap. There is a tendency to feel that you are in danger of becoming a vegetable. And, of course, you might. One way to lessen the danger is to continue to read and write. Remember the golden rules in the first chapter: read, read, read, write, write, write. Here are some reasons why you as a health professional might write articles:

- To publish a very good essay
- To express a point of view
- To share research findings
- To describe an innovative project
- To see your name in print
- To continue to enjoy the process of writing
- To earn some money.

Writing articles differs from writing essays. In this chapter we explore some of the technical details involved and examine the process of submitting work for publication.

Where to publish

Where you hope to publish your work depends on what sorts of article you intend to write. The following are examples of outlets for your work:

- Weekly magazines related to your field of the health professions
- Learned journals associated with your discipline
- Small 'fillers' for magazines
- A regular column in a weekly magazine.

The last two come in that order, as you are not likely to break into the fillers and regular column market until you have a considerable record of publishing in one or both of the first two. Writing articles for weekly magazines is different from writing papers for learned journals and the process of having your article dealt with by the publisher is different. Writing in the 1930s, Brande suggested the following:

> Have periodical debauches of book-buying and magazine-buying, and try to formulate to yourself the editor's possible requirements from the type of periodical he issues.
>
> Brande 1934

Writing for magazines

Most sections of the health professions have their own weekly or monthly magazines. In the nursing profession, for example, there are two weekly publications: the *Nursing Times* and the *Nursing Standard*.

Over to you

Find out what the main publications are for your health profession. Do they publish guidelines for potential contributors?

Weekly publications are usually looking for articles of between 800 and 2000 words in length. The sorts of article that are published vary but examples are:

- Short research reports
- Examples of good practice
- Historical articles
- Short, controversial pieces
- Case studies
- Discussions of current theory and practice debates.

The magazine that you have in mind may not accept articles 'on spec'. Some may only use in-house writers or commission articles from specialist writers. Some publish invitations to writers, and these are the easiest ones to judge in terms of the likelihood of your being able to write for them. If your magazine *does* publish such an invitation and it offers details of how to submit a manuscript, follow these to the letter. Do not assume that you can send in a manuscript that roughly follows them – make sure it is an exact fit. Do not risk rejection on the grounds that your manuscript was badly prepared.

If there is no such invitation, write a short letter to the editor, outlining the article that you have in mind. Keep the outline to one page of A4 and then wait until you have an answer. Some editors take a little while to respond. Do not worry them. If you have had no reply after about four weeks, try phoning the editorial department of the magazine. If you still get no response, write another letter to the editor. Be warned: editors vary in the amount of feedback they give you. Some send a standard, word-processed letter that has your name on it. Others will give you details of why they cannot accept your submission, if they turn it down. It is doubtful if many people will receive the sort of rejection slip that was published by a columnist in the *Financial Times*, who claimed it to be a genuine rejection slip from a Chinese economic journal:

> We have read your manuscript with boundless delight. If we were to publish your paper, it would be impossible for us to publish any work of a lower standard. And as it is unthinkable that in the next thousand years we shall see its equal, we are, to our regret, compelled to return your divine composition, and to beg you a thousand times to overlook our short sight and timidity.
>
> Findlater 1984

If you are asked to submit a manuscript or you have sent one to the editor, you will again have to wait some time to hear whether or not your work has been accepted. You may be asked to make modifications to the manuscript and the editor will give you detailed instructions as to how you can do this. On the other hand, your work may be edited in-house. There is no guarantee that the final published article will be exactly the same as your original submission. Also, you will be asked to sign away the copyright of your paper. While, with books, the author may continue to hold the copyright, with articles, the publisher owns it.

There may be a considerable delay between having your work accepted and seeing it in print. Sometimes the wait is up to one year.

One alternative way of seeing your name in print in some weekly magazines is to write short reports of research that you have carried out. These are usually about 250 to 500 words in length and contain details of your sampling, methodology and findings.

A thing you should never do is to send off a good essay that you have written for a course. Essays and published articles differ in important ways. First, you will have used the word 'essay' in your essay. Second, the style is likely to be rather 'academic'. The magazine article is likely to be in a 'snappier' style and illustrated with short case studies or examples from practice. Don't expect that a member of the editorial staff will rewrite your essay for you.

Some magazines will pay you for your work, and in this case you will receive payment after the article has been published. Rates vary from about £25 to £150. Most pay somewhere in between these two extremes. Some pay nothing at all.

About a month before publication, you will receive page proofs to check. The Society for Freelance Editors and Proofreaders can provide a useful guide as to the marks that you should use when correcting proofs. It is important to make a very clear statement here about correcting proofs:

Proofs are only for correcting – not for rewriting.

Changes in the text, at this stage, are very expensive. Make sure that all you do is correct typographical errors. Any other changes should have been ironed out before you sent in your manuscript. If you realise that you have made an important mistake and this has got through to page proofs, ring the editorial department of the magazine and talk through the problem with them.

Key points | Top tips

- Keep a record of any publications that you have. You will need to list these in your CV and publications will always enhance it.

Be careful about drawing illustrations for your article. While most magazines claim that you can send in 'rough drawings' for translation by their own artists, those artists cannot mind-read. You cannot expect them to 'know' what you really meant by lines in a diagram. Most will stick very closely to your original. If you draw an oval when you meant to represent a circle, the artist will draw an oval. It is a good idea to use simple drawing instruments to make sure that a diagram that you send in is as nearly exactly what you would like to see in the magazine as possible. Alternatively, ask the reprographics department of your college or university to draw the illustrations for you.

Once you have had a few articles published, you could ask the magazine if they would like some fillers. These are short pieces of between 200 and 500 words that the editorial staff can use to fill the bottoms of pages when other articles do not fit the page exactly. They give the opportunity to be controversial, to get something off your chest and to practise writing to deadline. You may be asked to write something at short notice and it is worth building up a small library of pieces that you could use in this way.

<table>
<tr><td>Key points</td><td>Top tips</td></tr>
</table>

- Read the Advice to Authors page, before you write an article for a journal
- Keep within the subject matter and word limit set by the journal
- Check everything, including the layout of your paper
- Be patient! Reviewing can take a long time.

After a while, you may also be asked to review other people's submissions and to comment on whether or not you feel the editor should publish a particular paper. Deal with this sort of request promptly – you are likely to be paid for the work. Also, be careful about what you write. Remember what it was like for *you* to receive criticism about your work. Treat people gently: egos are fragile, especially when they are attached to writing. Many people (and you may be one of them) finding writing very difficult. Do not be too ready to write off someone else's work. Do offer constructive comments on any manuscript you receive and do not simply write back with the comment 'This is OK, suggest you publish'. Make comments about why a piece should or should not be published and remember that the author is likely to be sent what you have written.

Writing for journals

The other sort of article writing is for academic journals. Some lecturers will want to concentrate almost exclusively on this sort of publication, for academic reputation is often based largely on the number of journal publications a person has. You may not agree with this state of affairs but it seems to be true. Certainly, in terms of CV development, journal articles will always 'score' higher than articles in magazines. This is reasonable, for journal articles are usually concerned with one or more of the following:

- Research reports
- Detailed searches of the literature
- Well argued, theoretical pieces.

Nearly all academic journals operate a blind refereeing system. That is to say, your submission will be sent to two peers in the field without their knowing your name. These referees will be asked to comment on whether or not your paper should be published. If it is not published but not turned down absolutely, you may be asked to rewrite part or the whole of your manuscript. Pay close attention to what you are being asked to do and make the changes quickly. When your manuscript is returned, it may be sent back to the referees for their opinion on your modified work.

There is a basic format for research-based papers. The following represent headings that you may want to follow in laying out your work.

- Abstract or summary
- Introduction
- Short literature review
- Aims of the study
- Methodology
- Findings
- Discussion
- Conclusions, including limitations of the study and implications for further research
- References.

As always, follow the 'Advice to Authors' that is usually printed inside the back page of the journal. Follow it to the letter. If the Advice asks you to double-space your manuscript, do not use one-and-a-half line spacing. If you are asked to submit three copies, make sure that you do. If you do not, it is quite likely that the editor will merely write to you to make the necessary modifications before even considering your work. You are unlikely to be paid for any contribution you make to an academic journal and you may have to wait up to a year to see your work in print.

As with other sorts of published work, you will be sent page proofs to correct. It is important that you read these only to make corrections and not to make modifications. Changes at this stage are very expensive and you will not be at all popular with the editor or the publisher if you try to make extensive alterations to the text.

One other thing that you should work at in relation to journal papers is to avoid sexist writing. Don't use 'man' when you mean 'person'. Avoid the generic use of 'man' as in 'mankind'. Also, avoid perpetuating professional stereotypes by automatically referring to nurses as she or to managers as he. On the other hand, don't get silly about it. Try to avoid really clumsy constructions such as 'personhole cover'.

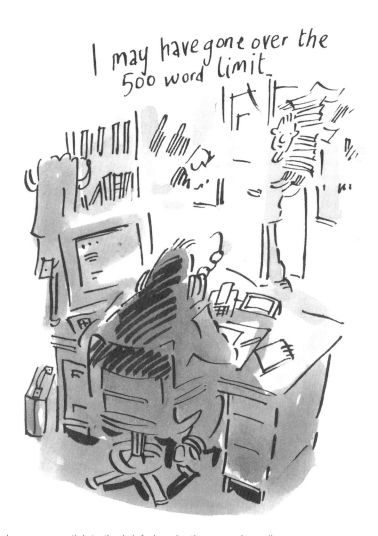

Make sure you stick to the brief given by the magazine editor.

Your aim is to communicate and not to offend. Nor is it your aim to draw attention to your writing by adopting a purposely odd style.

Spend some time in laying out your work. Avoid footnotes and endnotes wherever possible. Anything that is important enough to go into a footnote can be written into the body of the text. This comment is particularly relevant in these days of word processors. Perhaps, when people had to type their work, there was an excuse. To integrate a comment meant to retype the whole page, while a footnote could be added to the bottom of the page. Footnotes have gone out of fashion and few, I suspect, mourn their passing. Unfortunately, many of the larger commercial word-processing packages contain the necessary functions to create footnotes and some writers feel obliged to use them because they are there. Resist the temptation. Your paper will be better for your restraint and the editor will prefer it.

Top tips

- Avoid the temptation to pad out your work with high-flown sentence construction. Avoid such clichés as 'there is a sense in which' or 'it may be argued by some commentators that . . .'
- Try to write directly and to the point
- Keep your sentences short and also your paragraphs
- If you are writing a research report, stick to clear description. As I have indicated elsewhere, a student coming to your journal article should find enough information to set about a replication
- Read some of the early psychology and sociology reports as role models for clear writing. You may not agree with their research methods nor the ethics of some of their experiments. Often, though, their writing style is excellent.

Send your manuscript to one journal at a time. If it is rejected by one journal, send it to another. If it rejected by the second, reread it, adapt it and send it to a third. If the third rejects it, ask for candid comments from colleagues about ways in which you could improve or adapt it. Remember that some famous book manuscripts were rejected many times. So it is, sometimes, with academic journal manuscripts. Keep at it. You may have to: your job may depend on it.

One way to overcome the rejection problem is to co-write papers with people who already have a publication record. This can be a useful educational experience for both parties, for writing with another person means compromise. You cannot simply write what you like: you have to take into account what the other party feels. Be aware, though, that some university interview panels, when totting up publications, make a note of how many publications you have managed 'solo' and how many are joint publications. Avoid attaching your name to a long list of other people's. Try to write with one other person or on your own. This does not apply, of course, if you are part of a large research project in which it has been agreed that all of you will share publication authorship. It can all become rather clumsy, though and it may be better to divide the publications between you.

After you have had some journal papers published, you may feel brave enough to tackle a book. Again, you have the option, here, of the following:

- Writing the book yourself
- Writing it with one or two other people
- Editing a volume with chapters contributed by a number of people.

In my experience, the last often seems the most attractive but offers the hardest work (unless you really find writing difficult). Editing other people's prose is not easy. You have to be both rigorous and tactful. Such a balance is difficult to achieve and it is usually possible and easy to upset someone in the editing process. Also, with an edited volume, there is often a difference between what people tell you they will write and what they actually write. A worse possibility is that the person who told you they will contribute a chapter changes her mind. It happens, so be ready for it. All of this and more is discussed in the next chapter – about writing books.

RRRRRRapid recap

Check your progress so far by working through both the following questions.

1. Name two different types of article in your professional magazine.
2. What happens in a blind refereeing system?

If you have difficulty with either of the questions, read through the section again to refresh your understanding before moving on.

References

Brande, D. (1934) *Becoming a Writer*. Harcourt Brace, New York.

Findlater, R. (ed.) (1984) *Author! Author*! Faber & Faber, London.

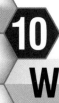

10 Writing books and reviews

Learning outcomes

By the end of this chapter you should be able to:

- Understand the important details to include in writing a book proposal
- Appreciate the basic clauses in a standard author contract
- Know the implications of copyright
- Structure and lay out a manuscript
- Prepare illustrations
- Understand the basic steps involved in book publishing.

Zest. Gusto. How rarely one hears these words used. How rarely do we see people living, or for that matter, creating by them. Yet if I were asked to name the most important items in a writer's make-up, the things that shape his material and rush him along the road to where he wants to go, I could only warn him to look to his zest, see to his gusto.

Ray Bradbury

That is what you have to have to write a book: zest and gusto. A book is like an article, only longer – considerably longer. All the rules of article writing apply to the writing of non-fiction books. And it is non-fiction that is discussed in this chapter. If you are planning to write a novel then you will have to look elsewhere for information.

Why should you want to write a book if you are a health professional? The reasons may be similar to article writing but there are some additional reasons. A short list might include:

- Because there is no book on the market that covers this particular aspect of the profession
- Because the profession needs a new book on the topic
- Because you have done research that you need to elaborate on
- Because you have an idea for a book that you think is a good one
- Because you like writing and want to write a book
- Because you have been approached by an editor
- Because you want to convey some of your own zest and gusto to other people.

There are no doubt numerous other reasons. Try to identify why *you* want to write a book. Also, consider the second to last reason in the list above. You need to *want* to write a book and not simply *like the idea*. While I suggested, a little fatuously, perhaps, that writing a book is a bit like writing an article, the point is that a book is much, much longer. You need to have stamina. As a starter, let's consider what an average non-fiction book comprises. Here is a fairly reasonable standard description:

- Between 50,000 and 100,000 words in length
- Between 10 and 12 chapters.

Put like that, it looks a bit daunting. Let us consider the lower end of the scale (and few editors or publishers will consider a manuscript less than 50,000 words in length). Supposing your book has 10 chapters. Then each chapter will be about 4500 words in length. The extra words will be taken up by appendixes, bibliographies and an introduction: all the words in the book count. Put like that, it may not seem so bad. Again, the keynote is structure. Nobody that I know sits down and starts from scratch, at page 1. The process of getting a idea for a manuscript also mitigates against such an approach. In the field of non-fiction, you don't write the book first. First, you have to have a contract from a publisher. That means two things. The publisher has to be behind your idea. Then, you have to write a detailed proposal about the sort of book you want to write. You may also be asked to write sample chapters. All this is good news for you. The process of preparing a proposal is the process of structuring a book. In this chapter, I will write in some detail about the planning of a proposal and working through that proposal.

The proposal

In essence, a book proposal is a book plan. It tells the editor that you have done some homework. You have surveyed the field, you have considered the opposition and you have a chapter-by-chapter plan of what you intend to write. You need to spend some time working on a proposal. After you have written it, you have to convince a publisher that it is worth their while publishing what you write.

How do you contact publishers? There are a number of routes. Here are a few:

- You ring up a publisher whom you know deals in works like the one you have in mind and ask for the name of the commissioning editor. Then you write a letter to that editor asking if she would read your proposal.
- You ring the commissioning editor directly and ask the same question. This is one of the best approaches. Ring the company first and find out the name of the commissioning editor, and then ring that person directly. It is usually best to work on a 'personal' basis in these matters.

- You talk to someone who has had a book published and you ask them to introduce you to a commissioning editor. You *may* get taken out for lunch by that editor but this is becoming a rare occurrence. I cannot remember the last time I was taken out for a meal by an editor, although some have threatened to.
- You are visited by an editor, at work. This happens quite often in university and college departments. Editors like to visit such places to try to persuade academics and their colleagues to submit proposals for books. I don't know what the success rate of this approach is.
- If you are an expert in your field, an editor may approach you to ask you to write a book.

Be prepared for a polite refusal and don't nag. The commissioning editor knows the field and knows what does and does not sell. If she really is interested, she will not risk letting your proposal getting away. If you are turned down first time, contact three or four other editors before you reconsider what might be wrong with your proposal. If possible, have someone who writes look through your plan with a critical eye. Then accept what they say and rewrite it. You have to be prepared to eat bowlfuls of humble pie in the book business. For that is what it is: a business. You will often be asked to rewrite. You will often find that your work is edited with a heavy hand. Accept this. If you don't, you will not get published. If you write a huge bestseller, then you might be able to ignore this advice. In the meantime, this is a case of doing as you are told. Publishers invest thousands of pounds in your proposal, if they accept it. It is they who call the shots. Mostly, too, they are right. They know what sells and what sits on shelves. You don't want your book to do the latter. Never believe people who say 'I just want to get a book published'. What they mean, as soon as they have had a proposal accepted, is 'I want to write a book that sells'.

It is important not to give up. If your idea for a book is good enough, it will be accepted for publication. Also, the better your

Key points Top tips

Just to recap, before identifying how to write a proposal:

- Make sure that you really do want to write a book and are not just in love with the idea
- Contact a publisher and get agreement to have your proposal read
- Accept the comments that the publisher makes, if they are interested in your proposal: if not, send it off to another
- Read any comments that the editor makes and incorporate them into a revamped proposal.

initial proposal – and the more detailed – the easier it will be to write. For the structure and detail of the proposal will give you a useful framework around which to base your book.

Writing a proposal

Most publishers mean the same sort of thing when they ask you for a proposal. They want a short document that identifies the following things:

- The name of the proposed book
- The author
- A rationale for the book
- The market
- Details about the author
- Comparison with other books in the field
- Contents
- Details of length, date of submission and so on.

Wells (1989) offers a useful checklist of things to think about when preparing a book proposal. He suggests, among other things, the following points:

- Have you clearly identified the target reader?
- Have you explained why the reader needs your book and how the reader will benefit from it?
- Have you explained why you are well qualified to write the book?
- Have you described your proposed book in the best possible terms?
- Have you covered the whole of the subject, or should you reduce the stated scope to match the coverage?
- Have you made clear that the book will meet all the requirements of the appropriate and specified examination syllabuses?
- Have you mentioned competitive books – and explained why yours will be better, or at least a valuable alternative?

Wells 1989

Wells's book, *The Successful Author's Handbook*, is an excellent guide to all aspects of writing non-fiction books and will be useful to anyone who is preparing to write one – for the first time or the 21st time.

I have decided that the best illustration of a book proposal would be one I have written (Figure 10.1 on page 148). It will, I hope, highlight better than detailed paragraphs the way a proposal looks when it is written. After you have read it through, I will share with you the editor's comments.

Book Proposal: Writing for Health Professionals
Philip Burnard PhD
Director of Postgraduate Nursing Studies, University of Wales College of Medicine, Cardiff

Rationale

Health professionals must write. Most need to continually update their education and training. Such courses call for essays, projects and dissertations. Health professionals working in colleges and university departments also need to publish. This book would offer a clear and direct guide to all types of writing: from essays to complete books. It would also deal with the question of using a computer to write – a topic that has been missing from many of the 'how to write' books.

Aims

- To provide a clear guide to all aspects of writing in the health professions

- To encourage health professionals to write

The book would be written in an easy-to-read style with full use made of bullet lists and checklists. Reference would be made to the relevant literature and a full bibliography offered at the end of the book. The overall aim would be a practical one: to help to get the health professional writing. The style would be in keeping with other books in the *Therapy in Practice* series.

Market

Students and trained staff in all the health and allied professions, including medicine, nursing, occupational therapy, physiotherapy and others. Educators, tutors and trainers in the health professions. Clinical and community-based practitioners.

The author

Director of postgraduate nursing studies, University of Wales College of Medicine, Cardiff and honorary lecturer in nursing, Hogeschool Midden Nederland, Utrecht, Netherlands. Author of 15 textbooks on communication, interpersonal skills training, counselling, research methods, ethics and education. Three titles published in the *Therapy in Practice* series and another in production. More than 130 published papers and articles in UK and USA. Manuscript and proposal reviewer for three British publishers, five health-care journals and book reviewer for four health-care journals. Masters degree in education and PhD in experiential learning.

Comparison with other titles

There are a number of general 'how to write' books on the market but these are mostly aimed at specific writing markets: the prospective author or the feature writer. The proposed book would be written especially for the health-care worker and would address a wider range of writing projects. The likely competitor in this field would be:

Turk, C. and Kirkman, J. 1989 Effective Writing: Improving Scientific, Technical and Business Communication: 2nd Edition: E. and F.N. Spon, London. This is a well-written and clear book about how to improve report and business writing. It addresses a different market from the new book.

The book

Words: 50,000
Line diagrams (Word illustrations): c 10
Other illustrations: none
Delivery of manuscript: 6 months from signing of contract or earlier

Contents

Introduction
- Who writes?
- Why write?

- What is in this book?
- How to use the book
- Writing and you

1. Writing: the basics
- Writing in the Health Professions
- Types of writing

Figure 10.1 *Example of a book proposal*

September 2001
Professor Philip Burnard

Figure 10.1 *Continued*

Was it accepted for publication without a struggle? Well, yes and no. First, it was reasonably suggested that, in a book of about 50,000 words, 16 chapters was far too many. I was asked, fairly quickly, to resubmit a new proposal in which I cut down the chapters to a more normal 10. Otherwise, the proposal was accepted by the publishing board. Incidentally, I sent back a new proposal by return of post. It is important to answer all queries and questions from publishers as quickly as possible. Publishers, like all businesses, work to a tight time schedule. If you want to see your book in print, don't keep them waiting. I don't want to sound like a 'yes' man on these issues but I have found it important and useful to work *with* publishers rather than arguing with them. As I have already suggested, they have published a few more books than you or I are likely to write. They are the experts in the book trade even if you are the expert in your particular field.

Some publishers ask you to complete a publishing proposal form rather than submit your own proposal – although no publisher is likely to reject, automatically, a well-written proposal laid out by a potential author. Such proposal forms usually ask the following questions and, clearly, they don't expect 'yes' or 'no' answers to the questions. If you can, have your answers typed into the form, although, oddly enough, this is becoming more difficult in the age of computers. It is often difficult to 'line up' your printer with sufficient accuracy to complete forms. I still keep a portable typewriter for filling in forms. The questions on the publisher's proposal form are likely to be variants of these:

- Your name and qualifications
- Your address and telephone number
- Present appointment
- Précis of career to date
- Previous publications
- Provisional title of the book
- Details of the subject of the proposed book
- A brief statement about the purpose of the book
- Why the book is needed
- Principal UK market for the book
- Other markets (USA, Europe, etc.)
- For which courses the book would be a required text
- For which courses the book would be one of a number of required texts
- For which courses the book would be supplementary reading

- Details of other professional staff who are likely to be interested in the book
- Competitive titles
- Advantages of your book over the above
- How quickly might the book become out of date?
- Approximate number of words required for the book
- Approximate number of illustrations required
- Time required to deliver final manuscript
- Names and address of people would be qualified to give an opinion of your work
- Any further information that might be useful.

What happens to a proposal when you send it to a commissioning editor? First, she reads it through and sees whether or not it would fit into the publishing house's plan and whether or not it is publishable and saleable. Then, if these criteria are satisfied, the proposal is sent to one or more reviewers, who are usually experts in the field, for their opinions. Like the editor, they recommend small or substantial changes to the proposal or may suggest that it is rejected altogether. In my experience, reviewers vary considerably in what they look for and what they write about proposals. Some publishers send the reviewers a standard assessment form. Some just ask for comments. Whatever the case, you will again have to bite your tongue and do what you are told. If you do not, it is likely that your book will not be published. This is not to say that you should become a publisher's doormat but merely to remind you that book publishing is a commercial venture. The publishers are not there to be astounded by your ideas and prose but to sell books.

Key points **Top tips**

- Break the writing of a book down into small tasks: prepare an outline of the whole thing and write small sections at a time
- Ask someone to read, critically, what you have written
- Check everything: spelling, grammar, word length, style, consistency, references, permissions to use other people's work.

You may or may not be sent the reviewer's comments to read. If you are, be prepared for something of a shock. Reading other people's comments about your work can be difficult. Most of us, I suspect, are fairly thin-skinned when it comes to criticism and criticism of written work – for reasons I do not understand – can be particularly painful. Not all reviewers bear in mind that the potential author might read their comments – although experienced ones do.

Not all reviewers pull their punches when it comes to describing how they feel about a particular proposal. I still get an odd feeling in the pit of my stomach when I open an envelope that I know contains a set of reviewer's comments about a proposal (or a completed manuscript). Don't get too concerned about it but be prepared.

If everyone is happy with your proposal, you will be sent a contract to write the book. **Do not begin writing until you have signed the contract.** This is important. The contract is your agreement with the publisher to write a particular book. It may not be the book that you started writing a year ago. Also, you may never get a contract at all. If this happens, it is unlikely that another publisher will be interested in a half-written or completed manuscript.

The contract

The contract that you sign with the publisher is an agreement, on your part, to write a particular book and on their part to publish it within a reasonable time limit. The clauses of a book contract are usually these:

- **The work**. Your manuscript, for the purposes of the contract, will be known rather quaintly as 'the work'. In this clause, the agreed title will be used. The title is not binding and you or the editor may agree to use another one at a later date. Incidentally, titles are not copyright. In theory, you are free to write books called *Gone With the Wind* or *Alice in Wonderland*, although I don't recommend it.

- **Rights granted**. This is a statement that the publisher will have sole and exclusive right and licence to produce and publish your work. The copyright remains yours.

- **Delivery of the work**. This is a time limit for the delivery of the completed manuscript.

- **State of the typescript**. This spells out that you have both agreed a format for the typescript.

- **Illustrations**. This identifies your and the publisher's responsibility for supplying illustrations for your work.

- **Permissions**. This refers to your responsibility for obtaining permission to quote directly from other people's published work. Normally, under the 'fair dealing' agreement, you are able to quote short passages from other people's work without written permission. If in doubt, contact the editor.

- **Editing the typescript**. This clause conveys the publisher's right to edit your work into a house style acceptable to both parties.
- **Publisher's undertaking**. This is a formal statement that, everything else being equal, the company will publish your book.
- **Author's warranty**. This is the clause that says that the publisher will defend your copyright.
- **Warnings in the text**. This clause acknowledges that, if you are going to recommend dangerous exercises or activities, you will publish a warning with them.
- **Liability for author's property**. This clause is a let-out clause for the publisher. It states that they are not insured against their losing your work. Make sure you keep copies and ask for an acknowledgement of receipt of your manuscript.
- **Competing works**. Reasonably, you are asked not to write a competing book during the time of your agreement with the company.
- **Moral rights of author**. This asserts that the work is yours and will be published under your name and that you can object to the way in which your work has been treated by the publisher.
- **Royalties**. This clause spells out what, if any, royalties you will be paid. For example it could be 10% of the cover price per copy, or 10% of the company's net receipts from the sales of the book.
- **Subsidiary rights**. This clause is about the publisher's rights to sell your work to other companies or to sell the film rights. This clause is unlikely to affect your non-fiction book.
- **Accounts**. Here, the publisher tells you how often the company will pay you royalties. At the moment, some companies pay twice yearly, others yearly. The trend is towards once-yearly payment.
- **Examination of accounts**. Here, you are told that you can examine the company's accounts as they relate to your work. I have yet to meet anyone who has challenged a publisher on this issue but bear in mind that all publishers send you a thorough breakdown of your sales every time they send you a royalties cheque.
- **Presentation copies**. This clause tells you how many free copies you will be given when the book is published and at what discount you can buy further copies. Go easy with your free copies when you receive them. I once worked with a publisher that gave me 25 free copies (3 to 6 is normal) and I handed them out to all and sundry thinking the supply would last forever. I was down to two copies within a fortnight. In the excitement of receiving your free copies, it is easy to get carried away. It is a good idea to hold back at least 3 copies for your own use.

One for your bookshelf. One to show or lend to your friends (and which can be allowed to get dog-eared) and a third copy as a 'spare'. The third copy might be useful as a present for someone later on, when all the fuss has died down. Don't forget, too, that every book you give away means the potential loss of a sale. If you give someone your book, they do not have to buy it.

- **New editions**. This is about your being asked to produce a second and subsequent editions if the book sells well. Normally, you will only be asked to prepare a second edition after the first has sold well for about five years. Don't confuse printings with editions. Your book, if it sells well, may be reprinted as it stands. After five years you may be asked to update and/or partially rewrite your book. This will be the second edition.

- **Termination**. This outlines the limits to your relationship with the publisher and the grounds for cancelling the agreement.

- **Notice**. This tells you how to terminate the agreement.

- **Arbitration**. This is an important clause. It points out that the agreement is binding under English law and explains how any dispute may be arbitrated.

- **Advance**. This clause tells you how much money the company will pay you in advance of publication and when.

Read your contract carefully. If you have any doubts about clauses in the contract, contact the publisher for clarification. If you write books regularly and work with a variety of publishers, you may want to consider joining the Society of Authors. You can do this once you have had one full-length book published, for an annual subscription. The Society offers a book contract reading and vetting service and it is a very prompt and thorough one. Mostly, though, contracts are fairly standard, along the lines of the clauses discussed above. One clause that may be in your contract and one that you might want to query is one that says that the publisher will have first refusal on your next book. This is rather limiting if you do not want to write exclusively for one publisher. If you do not want to be bound by it, talk to the editor and then strike out the clause. Your signature of the contract will require a witness. Once you have signed the contract you are bound by it.

Key points Top tips

Don't skip the thorough reading of a book contract. It will contain many clauses that will affect the way in which your book is published, what royalties you earn and many other aspects of publishing. If you are not sure about an aspect of the contract, check it with the publisher

Advances

Some publishers will allow you an advance on royalties as an incentive. This can take a number of forms:

- A single amount following the signing of contracts. I have found this amount to vary from £100 to £700. Forget any ideas that you will be offered millions.
- An amount following the signing of contracts and an amount on the delivery of an acceptable manuscript.
- A single amount following the acceptance of a suitable manuscript. Note the words 'an acceptable manuscript'. That means acceptable to the publisher. You may be asked to rewrite sections or chapters before you see your advance.
- An amount on publication of the book.

Some publishers give no advances at all. There is one important thing to remember: an advance is just that. What you are paid prior to publication will have to be paid back from the royalties that you earn once the book is published. Therefore, it is wise not to push for high advances (unless you are really broke). If you do, it may be some time before you see any other earnings from your work.

A few academic imprints give you no royalties at all. They publish research monographs for small markets and you have to submit camera-ready copy of your manuscript. That is to say that the copy you submit is the copy that will appear in the finished book. The publisher undertakes to publish your work quickly and to give you a certain number of free copies. Such books are usually hard-bound for sales to libraries and universities. You will not make any money but you will see your work in print in a short space of time. This sort of publishing is useful if you want to pass on your PhD findings to a larger audience. Few other types of publisher will publish theses as they stand. Some will ask for a major rewrite, which you may not want to do. Others will not be interested at all. This sort of publishing enterprise offers a useful service to academics and researchers who might otherwise have to rely only on journal publications.

One sort of publishing to avoid is vanity publishing. This is a form of publishing where you pay for everything. The publisher agrees to help you publish your book but you pay for all aspects of the process from reading the manuscript to having the book printed. Most vanity publishers do little to promote their authors and most bookshops will not stock books from vanity publishers. The net result could be that you are stuck with a garage full of unsaleable books. Don't do it. If you book is worth publishing, a 'real' publisher will publish it.

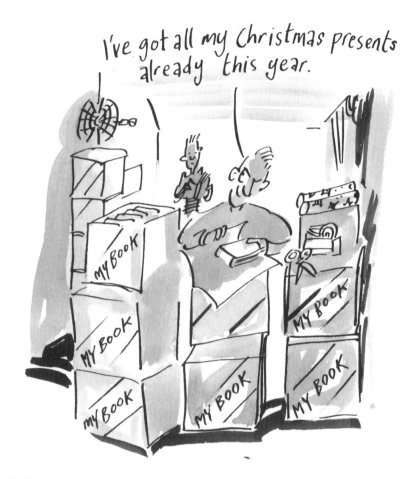

Vanity publishing will probably mean you have to literally give your book away.

Writing the book

There are various things to say about writing a book. These, like other aspects of writing, can be divided into stages:

- Completing the outline
- Doing the research
- Doing the writing
- Preparing the manuscript
- Sending it to the publisher
- Waiting
- Dealing with queries, the author's questionnaire and proof-reading
- Preparing the index.

Completing the outline

First, the proposal must be worked upon. All the headings and subheadings need to be broken down further into manageable and writable chunks. It is a good idea, at this stage, to allocate words to each section and to try to stick to those word limits.

Doing the research

You are unlikely to have enough knowledge in your head to complete the book in one go. This means, rather like writing essays, you must make many trips to the library for references, books and journal papers. Then, you need to file them away in such a way that you both remember them and can find them quickly. Some people have elaborate filing systems. I tend to work in the middle of a pile of papers and books and can usually find what I want. Information for new books can be gleaned from a number of sources. Here are a few:

- Research carried out by the writer
- Other people's research reports
- Public and college libraries
- Journal papers and articles
- Life experience
- Your own experience of the health profession
- Interviews.

Doing the writing

Get into a writing habit. If you can, write every day and do not stop until you have reached the target that you have set yourself. You do not have to write the book straight through. Start with a chapter you feel confident about and write that first. On the other hand, do not leave the most difficult chapter until last. Try to end on an easy chapter too. Keep an eye on three things:

- Accuracy
- Consistency of style
- Simplicity.

Again, resist the urge to be long-winded or clever. You may be writing 50,000 words but every one has to count. You cannot pad out a book any more than you can pad out an essay. If you do, it is unlikely that people will read it. Most people can spot 'page filling' a mile off.

If at all possible, write straight into a word-processing program on a computer. This will allow you all sorts of control over the writing and editing process. Write first, fairly quickly. Then go back and edit what you have written.

Copyright

There is sometimes confusion in people's minds about the question of copyright. You do not have to register or publish a piece of written work in order for it to be considered copyright. The fact that you have written it at all means that you already own the copyright to the work. Note, though, that when you sell an article to a publisher, you are often asked to sign over the copyright of the piece to that publisher. This means, in effect, that the publisher can do what it likes with your piece. The publisher may edit it significantly and may sell it on to other publishers without, legally, having to tell you. In practice (we hope) most publishers of journals will tell you that they are selling your work to other publishers. In one case, though, I had the experience of opening an American book – in order to review it – only to find that the book contained a chapter made up of an article I had had published in a British journal some years before. Clearly, the journal had sold the piece on, but without telling me. How widespread this practice is, it is difficult to say but it is to be hoped that it happens fairly rarely.

In the case of book publication, the author usually retains the copyright. If you look at the reverse of the title page of most books, you will see that the author's name stands next to the copyright sign © – an indicator that the author still holds the copyright. Incidentally, there is no need to use the copyright sign in documents that you produce for other purposes (e.g. reports, curriculum documents, brochures etc.). As we have seen, the writer of these automatically holds the copyright by virtue of having written the document.

On rare occasions, a publisher may ask an author to sign over copyright to that company. In this case, you may want to consider very carefully whether or not this is something you are prepared to do.

Sometimes, you will want to quote other people's work directly in your own book. The copyright law is far from specific on the question of how much or how little you can do this but one thing is certain: you *must* acknowledge your sources. You must indicate when a piece of writing has been quoted directly from other people's work. Not to do this constitutes plagiarism and legal action can follow such a breach of copyright. The usual format for indicating direct quotations from other people's work is to indent the paragraph containing the quote and to offer, in brackets, the original author's name and the year of publication (in the text) and the full reference to the work from which the quote was taken (in the reference list at the back of the book or at the end of the chapter).

Barry Turner (1992) offers a useful summary of the general principles of quoting from other people's work as follows:

> The rule is, a writer has the undisputed right to quote another writer for 'purposes of criticism or review', as long as 'sufficient acknowledgement' is given. There are limits of course. It is not the done thing to lift a 'substantial part' of a copyright work without permission. Unfortunately, there is little agreement on what constitutes 'a substantial part'. . . . Common sense suggests basing the assessment on the length and importance of the quotation; the amount quoted in relation to the text as a whole; the extent to which the work competes with the work quoted, and the extent to which the words quoted are saving a writer time and trouble.
>
> Some years ago, the Society of Authors and The Publisher's Association stated that they would usually regard as 'fair dealing' the use of a single extract of up to 400 words or a series of extracts (of which none exceeds 300 words) to a total of 800 words from a prose work, and extracts to a total of 40 lines from a poem, provided that this did not exceed a quarter of the poem.
>
> Turner 1992

Bear in mind that when you do quote from other people's work, you must quote exactly what is written in the original text – including the original punctuation. If you leave out a small section of the text, you indicate this with an ellipse (. . .) as indicated in the above quotation. If you want to emphasise something of the original text, you do so by placing the words in italics and at the end of the quotation you add the following, in brackets: *emphasis added*. As we have seen, it is not good practice to use the term 'sic' after a quotation to show that you have spotted a grammatical error. If the quotation was that bad, it was probably better not to use it at all. Incidentally, if the passage does contain a grammatical, typographical or spelling error, you must not 'correct' this. Instead, you still write out the quotation exactly as it appeared in the original publication. Again, though, you may want to consider whether or not you use such a quotation.

Sometimes, a publisher will ask you to obtain 'permission' from the publisher of the original text, for use of the quotation(s). In this case, your publisher may supply you with 'permission forms'. In this case, you fill in the form as a request to the second or subsequent publishers to ask permission to quote from their books. Those publishers, if they are happy for you to use the quotation(s), will then stamp the form, indicating that permission has been granted. In some cases – particularly when the quotation is a 'literary' or poetic one, there may be a charge for the use of a quotation. Also, of course, permission may *not* be granted, although, in practice, this is rare.

It should be noted that no one holds the copyright to book titles. Thus, if you publish a book called *Legal Aspects of Health Care Work*, there is nothing to stop another author writing a book by the same title. In choosing your own title, though, it is probably best to do some homework. It is not, generally, good practice to 'borrow' someone else's title. After all, your buyer may end up purchasing the other writer's book and you have lost a sale.

Copyright normally lasts for 70 years from the end of the calendar year in which the author dies. This rule applies to unpublished as well as published work.

Preparing the manuscript

Once you have written the manuscript, you need to make sure that it is in a fairly standard format before you send it to the publishers. Publishers rarely seem to tell you what they want but experience suggests that there are certain rules of layout for a manuscript submission. They are these:

- Print on one side of good-quality A4 paper.
- Double-space the lines.
- Leave good margins around the edge of your work (about 3.5 cm on all sides).
- Put numbers on all pages and number the manuscript consecutively from the first page to the last. Don't start again at 1 for a new chapter. If you need to insert a page before sending off the manuscript, call the new pages 26b . . . 26c, etc. If there are a number of extra pages, renumber the entire manuscript. Don't forget that your word processor can automatically number the pages for you. I put the number at the bottom of the page, in the centre. I have read that some

publishers prefer page numbers in the top right hand corner. I have not had any complaints.

- Don't use 'headers' or 'footers'. Your aim is not to produce a manuscript that looks like a book but one on which the copy-editor can work. She will not thank you if she has to cross out headers and footers on every page.

- Don't use a wide range of fonts. Stick to a standard 12-point font throughout.

- Print diagrams on separate pages and don't integrate them with the text. Put the diagram next to the page to which it refers.

- Don't bind the manuscript at the side. Do not staple it but leave the pages free.

- At the top of each page, print your name and the title of the manuscript. This is just in case anyone drops part of it and then wonders to which pile of papers these particular ones refer.

Figure 10.2 illustrates one page of manuscript from this chapter as I submitted it to the publisher. It illustrates a number of the issues identified in the above list. Notice, too, the indentations that break up the text into paragraphs. There is never an indent at the beginning of a piece of text, under a subheading. The paragraphs following, however, are indented.

Then, if these criteria are satisfied, the proposal is sent to one or more reviewers, who are usually experts in the field, for their opinions. Like the editor, they make recommend small or substantial changes to the proposal or may suggest that it is rejected altogether.

In my experience, reviewers vary considerably in what they look for and what they write about proposals. Some publishers send the reviewers a standard assessment form. Some just ask for comments. Whatever the case, you will again have to bite your tongue and do what you are told. If you do not, it is likely that your book will not be published.

That is not to say that you should become a publisher's doormat but merely to remind you that book publishing is a commercial venture. The publishers are not there to be astounded by your ideas and prose but to sell books.

Advances

Some publishers will allow you an advance on royalties as an incentive. This can take a number of forms:

- An amount following the signing of contracts and an amount on the delivery of an acceptable manuscript.

75

Figure 10.2 *Example of a page of book manuscript*

The preparation of illustrations

Illustrations are attractive but they are also expensive. Remember that if you want to use other people's pictures, photographs or diagrams you will have to obtain permission to do so. You are likely, too, to be asked by the publishers to supply these illustrations in a format that will allow the printers to print direct from the material that you supply. This, again, can be an added expense.

Photographs, particularly those containing people, can 'date' very easily. Hairstyles and lengths change more quickly and so do styles in glasses and clothes. Try to avoid, particularly, photographs that do not really illustrate any particular point. These are the sort that bear legends such as 'a group of students enjoying working together' or 'many nurses work in the community' and accompany pictures of groups of people doing nothing in particular. This is an expensive way of filling pages.

Simple line illustrations are possibly the most inexpensive choice if you have to have illustrations. They consist of black and white diagrams of a fairly rudimentary nature. 'Box' diagrams that draw attention to particular points also fall into this category. Remember that the diagrams you send in with your manuscript must be a very accurate representation of what you want to see on the printed page. You cannot assume that the publisher's graphics department can 'guess' what you had in mind. If you send in a diagram of particular proportions, you are likely to find that the proofs you receive echo those proportions. Remember, too, that changes to line diagram proofs can be very expensive. So keep the diagrams simple and make sure that they are accurate. If you feel unable to draw sufficiently good diagrams yourself, enrol a friend or colleague to work on them. Some colleges and universities have a 'graphics department' that can also help. The *Nelson Thornes Author Guide* (2003) offers the following directions about line illustrations to their authors:

- As you write the text, produce detailed rough versions or detailed written notes for each illustration, preferably separate from your script (with some indication on the script of your preferred position for the item and any flexibility in positioning).
- Try to state which type of illustration you require and its precise content. Where possible provide references to support your instructions.
- You should also provide captions for your illustrations.
- Draw your roughs at the size you want them (or larger if there is a lot of detail, then specify a final ideal size for reproduction). Indicate clearly which parts of the artwork require labels.

Sending it to the publishers

When you are quite sure that the manuscript is complete and you have checked the spelling, ensured that all pages are numbered and printed out a clean copy, you are ready to send it off to the publisher. If you have no other instructions, send two copies: the top copy and a photocopy. Also, keep a hard copy for yourself. Don't rely on the copy you have on disk. If the editor rings up and asks about something on page 38, it will be difficult to find that page if all the chapters exist only as computer files.

A medium-sized manuscript is best packed in a padded posting bag, well sealed. Enclose a letter outlining what is in the package and post it off. If the manuscript is too large for this, send it in the box that the paper was packed in. It is a good idea to enclose a self-addressed card to enable the publishers to acknowledge receipt of the manuscript. I have sent off a manuscript and waited for over 2 weeks to hear whether or not it was received. When I phoned the publisher, they told me that they had received it 10 days previously. There is no guarantee that publishers will automatically acknowledge receipt, so make it easy for them.

Presentation of manuscripts on disk

The completed manuscript must also be sent on disk or e-mailed as attached files. This speeds up production of your book and can save production costs. You may be invited to respond to editors' comments by reference to either the disk version of your manuscript or the printed version.

If you are planning to send in your manuscript on disk, there are certain rules that you must follow. These include the following:

- Use a standard, well-known word-processing program and tell the publishers which one you have used. This is usually discussed in advance of your sending in your work.
- Create a separate file for each chapter and for other sections of the book such as the introduction, preface, bibliography and so on. Give these files readily recognisable names (e.g. CHAP1.DOC, BIBLIOG.DOC).
- Keep illustrations in separate files and name them clearly.
- Keep files reasonably small (about 100 kb is the maximum). If your chapters are larger than this, divide them into two and name them appropriately (e.g. CHAP1A.DOC, CHAP1B. DOC).

- Be consistent in your layout and keep the layout very simple. Use one font throughout, if possible and indicate headings and subheadings in the same font. Keep headings and subheadings to the left hand margin and do not centre text.
- Don't attempt to design or lay out the final product. Keep your files as simple text files as far as is possible.
- Don't include diagrams, lines or boxes in the body of the text.
- Avoid footnotes as far as possible. This is good, general writing practice.
- Don't put in 'hard returns' at the ends of lines. In other words, don't press the 'enter' or 'return' key at the end of each line but allow the text to 'word-wrap'.
- Use the following codes within your text to indicate chapter headings, headings and subheadings:

  <<CN>>   in front of a chapter heading

  <<A>>   in front of major headings within chapters

  <<B>>   in front of the next level of subheading

  <<C>>   in front of sub-subheadings.

- As far as possible, avoid any further levels of subheading.
- Wherever possible, avoid using underlining. Instead, use italics and use those sparingly. Again, this is good general writing practice. As far as possible, avoid using underlining in any manuscripts. Underlining is 'shorthand' for italics and was used on typewriters before italicisation was possible.

Some academic publishers will accept your manuscript on disk as camera-ready copy and, if this is so, it will have been discussed with you. If you submit a manuscript in this format, bear in mind your responsibility. The printers will use your disk directly in the process of printing out the pages of your book. Any mistakes in the layout or typography of the text will be reproduced in the book itself. This is in contrast to the advice and information given in the previous paragraphs. It should be emphasised that most publishers will modify your text on disk quite considerably before your book is printed. If you *do* have to submit camera-ready copy on disk, you must spend a lot of time on making sure that the file on the disk exactly matches the way you want your text to appear on the printed page. If it is at all possible, avoid agreeing to submit text in this way. On the other hand, as we have seen, the supply of unformatted text – as described above – can help speed up the production of your book and keep costs down. This, in turn, may help keep down the cover price of your book and may well mean that you sell more copies.

Waiting

Then the wait. There is usually a considerable time gap between sending off the completed manuscript and hearing anything from the publisher. The temptation is strong to ring and find out what is happening. Do this if it makes you feel better but be assured that the process of book publishing is a fairly slow one. Also, be warned that people in the publishing field tend to change jobs with alarming frequency. You may not finish your book with the editor you started with.

The first thing you are likely to hear from the publisher is the satisfying sound of your advance on royalties cheque plopping on to the door mat. After that, another long silence.

During this period, the following things are happening at the publishers:

- The editor may read the manuscript to see whether or not it is in line with what was expected
- The editor will certainly ask one of the reviewers to read it and comment on it
- During this period, the editor will send for estimates of printing costs. There is a narrow and small profit margin on non-fiction books.

After these things have happened, the editor may write back to you with suggested modifications or rewrites. Do them and do them quickly. Time is all-important now, for time, at this stage, is money.

Once a complete and satisfactory manuscript is with the publisher, the next stage is that the manuscript is sent to a copy-editor who laboriously works through the entire manuscript checking on the spelling, style, grammar, sentence construction, references and just about everything else in the book.

Jill Baker, in a useful book about copy-editing, suggests the following advice to copy-editors about three levels on which to read and correct manuscripts:

1. Word by word, for consistency and conformity to style, correct spelling and syntax, inclusion of complete and correct references to bibliography and illustrations, accuracy of information as far as you know.
2. Sentence by sentence and paragraph by paragraph for clarity and succinctness. If you have to read a sentence twice in order to understand it, then it needs to be changed. You should also be alert to the possibility of libel.
3. Section by section and chapter by chapter for sense. You are looking to ensure that the author's arguments are cogent,

continuing and finally conclusive, that he does not introduce a new idea or character and then abandon it or him unresolved. In other words that the book hangs together as a complete work

Baker 1987

Copy-editors are the unsung heroes of the book trade. A good one can transform a mediocre manuscript into a reasonably good one but rarely gets any acknowledgement for it. The copy-editor has the difficult task of making sure that your book conforms to the publisher's 'house style' and is intelligible. On the other hand, she also has to retain the author's own style and approach to writing. Her aim is not to mechanically reduce every manuscript to a pre-determined format. If your book is well copy-edited, write and thank the copy-editor.

Dealing with queries, the author's questionnaire and proof-reading

After the copy-editor has worked carefully through your manuscript, she will have put together a list of queries about your work. This will usually take the form of conflicting dates of references in the text and in the list at the end, unclear phraseology or (if you are lucky) queries about the accuracy of some of the statements you have made. Again, deal with these quickly but make sure that your answers are fully made and that you make it absolutely clear what you mean. Writing 'OK' next to a query is not sufficient: you must make it completely obvious what you are saying OK to.

This is the last chance you have to make modifications to your manuscript. You cannot make changes at proof stage. If you really must make changes, make them now. Don't expect the copy-editor to be pleased with you. Changes should have been made before you submitted the manuscript.

Be considerate of the copy-editor's queries. Sometimes a point that is obvious to you is queried by the copy-editor. She is unlikely to be an expert in your particular field. If a point is not clear to the copy-editor it is unlikely to be clear to the general reader of your book. Bear in mind, though, that the copy-editor is the expert in editing. Read through any proposed changes carefully and do not dismiss them lightly. I have nearly always found that copy-editors improve on the original text. Figure 10.3 shows an example of a set of copy-editor's queries and the author's response to them.

About this time, too, you will be sent an 'author's questionnaire'. This will ask you a whole range of questions about your book. You

Smith & Davies Ltd
EDITORIAL QUERY SHEET
TITLE: Developing Professional Skills   AUTHOR: Edwards, J.

QUERY From copy-editor	REPLY/COMMENT from author
p24. 'Professions': should this be 'Professionals'?	Yes
p36. Lain: should this be Latin?	Yes
p67. 'of' in question: is this right? Should it be 'for'?	Yes, it should be 'for'.
p98. 'Indifference': should this be 'indifferent'?	Yes
p125. 'can perhaps . . . rather than . . .': is a word missing here?	Yes, please insert 'hinder'
p240. Cooper reference: no journal title	Journal title is Nurse Educator
p300. Brown (1994): Initial missing	Initial is J.
p302. Moore, Bianchi-Gray and Stevens: no initial for Stevens	Initial is P.
p305. Yardley and Honess (1987): not in refs	Yardley, K. And Honess, T. (Eds) (1987) Self and Identity, Wiley, Chichester.
p303. Smith and Cassen (1986): 1987 in refs	1987 is correct
p45. Saunders, not Owen in refs.	Saunders is correct.
p67. Peters 1976, 1969: 1972 in refs	1976 is correct. Please adjust 1969 ref and remove 1973 ref.
p79. Andrews 1958: 1957 in refs	1958 is correct
p.128. Brown 1989: 1981 in refs	1989 is correct
p230. Johns, 1993: a or b?	'a' is correct
p268. Shaffer 1978: Shafer in refs.	Shaffer is correct
p260. Whittaker (or Whitaker over page) 1987: not in refs	Whitaker, D.S. (1987) Using Groups to Help People, Tavistock/Routledge, London.

Figure 10.3 *Example of a set of copy-editor's queries*

will be asked, for example, to describe the book in a sentence, a short paragraph and to list the aims of the book. Spend considerable time filling this in carefully. The information gleaned from this questionnaire helps the publisher to brief sales staff and to sell your book. It may be tedious (and, for some reason, it almost always is) but do it well. Again, do it quickly. The author's questionnaire nearly always follows the following format and it is worth considering, in advance, what your answers to some of the questions might be. The more time you investing in working through these questions, the better the publishers will be able to market your book. Don't skimp on it. The items in a typical questionnaire are these – and I have added comments on them:

- **Title of the book**.

- **Your name, qualifications and affiliations**. Note that this will be used as text in promotional material. Decide beforehand whether or not you want all your qualifications next to your name or whether or not you want to be associated directly with your place of work. If you work in a large college, do you want to be associated, mostly, with the college, itself, or – more specifically – with the department within that college?

- **Your nationality and date of birth**. These are required for the registration of your book's copyright.

- **Home and work addresses and telephone numbers**. In this section, the publisher usually asks you which point of contact you would prefer. If you possibly can, quote an e-mail address or fax number in this section to allow the editor to get in touch with you quickly.

- **Career and present position**. Many publishers ask for a listing of work experience in the format of a short CV. Some, too, ask you to describe yourself in a fairly short paragraph. Don't be over-modest in this section. Again, the text may appear in advertising material. Obviously, though, do not make false claims about yourself.

- **Previous publications**. List here any other books, journal papers or articles that you have had published.

- **Description of the book**. Now the fun starts. In this section, you are normally asked to describe your book in about 250 words. You are required to say something about the purpose, aims, scope and general approach of the book. Again, choose your words carefully – and note the next section.

- **Description of your book in a few sentences**. This is the condensed version and often the most difficult to write. This and the previous section are two of the most important items in the questionnaire. Take your time over them.

- **What are the key features of your book?** You may be having a sense of *déjà vu* at this point. You may feel that you have said all that you can about your book in the previous sections. Here, though, you are required to supply a 'bullet list' (*this* is a bullet list) of the most important features that differentiate your book from others. If there is something really new or different about your book, this is the place to say it. These points often appear on the back cover of your book as part of the blurb. Remember that readers often read the back cover when trying to decide whether or not to buy your book. Remember, too, next time you read the back of someone else's book, that they probably wrote the back cover as well as the inner contents!

- **New edition**. If this is a second or subsequent edition of your book, you are asked here to identify in what ways the new edition is different.

- **Competition**. In this section, you are asked to identify the most important – in your view – competitors in the book market. Here, you compare your book with others and make sure that the publishers know that yours is the best one on the market. The information from this section is often used by sales representatives selling your book to booksellers. Be accurate about the competition but also make sure you 'sell' your own.

- **Superiority over other books**. This is where the publisher almost calls your bluff. You have to justify why your book is better than others. Again, you may feel that you have already done this but this is the opportunity to really identify the differences between your book and all the others. Do this well.

- **Weaknesses of other texts**. The publisher allows you your own back. Identify here the things that make the other books in the field less saleable than yours.

- **Readership**. In this section you identify, as clearly as possible, the groups of people that are likely to buy your book. Before you fill this section in, read the next.

- **Course texts**. Here, you describe what, if any, courses your book is appropriate for. You need to be accurate here as you are asked to *name* the courses that you have in mind. Be specific. No one benefits from your writing 'all courses for health professionals' in this section. You may need to do some research to fill in this – and the previous section – properly.

- **Countries**. If you feel that your book would sell well in other countries, this is your chance to list them. It is worth discussing with the editor whether or not there really is likely to be a market in other countries for your book. Do not guess at it and, again, do not use vague statements like 'all English-speaking countries'.

- **Reviews**. In this section you list the journals in which your book might be reviewed. The publishers will use your list (and its own) to make decisions about which journals should receive a free copy of your book for review purposes. Note that this does not in any way guarantee that your book *will* be reviewed in those journals. Book editors of journals receive huge numbers of books and reviewers often take huge amounts of time over the writing of reviews. You will probably find that you take much less time to review other people's books once you have had one of your own published. You can also list overseas journals in this section. Again, be specific and be realistic. You are unlikely to get a popular book about making friends reviewed in the *British Medical Journal* – although you might.

- **Professional societies**. Here you list any organisations, associations, unions and so on that might help to promote your book.

- **Conferences and exhibitions**. In this section, you identify any conferences at which you are likely to be presenting papers or any exhibitions in which you may feature. Sometimes, too, you are asked to list individuals who might be sent a free copy of your book. Identify these people really carefully and don't include your mother. Well-placed, free copies can help to sell your book.

- **Any other points**. In this final section, you are asked to identify any suggestions you may have for promoting your book. Once again, be realistic but do write down what you feel can be done. Unless your book is considered to be a major textbook, it is unlikely that it will be very widely advertised on its own. It will, of course, be included in the publisher's catalogues and you may like to ask for some 'flyers' so that you can engage in a bit of self-promotion. Undue modesty rarely pays. Books have a limited bookshelf life and you may as well promote your own books as hard as you can for the life that they do have. You may not be able to send everyone you can think of a copy of your book but you could certainly send them a flyer about it. You can also include these with some of your correspondence – both home and overseas.

Finally, you will be sent one or two copies of the proofs when they are printed. Normally, you will receive page proofs. These are rough prints of the pages of your book and will show you what the finished product will look like. I always enjoy opening parcels of page proofs.

If you are making an index, one of the copies of the proofs is for you to use in doing that. The other set is for proof-reading.

Making an index

Making an index is considered by many to be something of an art. It probably is. The good indexer anticipates the sorts of thing that people are going to look up and is restrained enough not to make the list so huge that it puts the user off. A good index can be really useful. A poor one is worse than no index at all. Two examples come to mind. First, the index that accompanies Turner's *The Writer's Handbook* is an example to anyone who plans to develop an index. On the other hand, the index to Reason and Rowan's *Human Inquiry: a sourcebook of new paradigm research* (a book that is excellent in every other respect) illustrates how not to produce an index. In that book, the word 'act' is referenced to 171 page numbers while the word 'analysis' is cited 110 times. It is fairly unlikely that many people would want to look up the word 'act' and even less likely that anyone would want to check it that number of times.

There are indexers whose full time job it is to make indexes. There are books on the topic, there are associations of indexers and even journals on indexing. In this section, I describe how *I* make an index. I have indexed most of the books that I have written and don't claim that they are examples of the state of the art. However, the method that I describe here does work.

Bear in mind that although your word-processing program is likely to have an indexing feature, you are unlikely to be able to use it at this stage. Remember that you are working with proofs supplied by the publisher. Indexing features in word processors work to the page numbers of the files that are produced within those word processors. The page numbers in proofs will be different to those in your files. Therefore, you have little option but to make your index by hand. Here is how I do it. The method, incidentally, is based to some degree on a reading of the books about indexing and to some degree on 'making it up as I went along'. I remember that, for a long time, I could not work out at all how to make an index: the task seemed gargantuan and I couldn't imagine where anyone started the process. Like most things, though, indexing becomes easier (and more obvious) as you start to do it.

First, though, some preliminaries. You don't need to index every word in your book. Clearly, no one is likely to want to look up 'the' or 'that'. But nor are they likely to look up the word 'counselling' in a book about counselling. After all, the *book* is about counselling. To index every occurrence of the word 'counselling' would produce huge numbers of page entries. And this leads to the second point: limit your entries. It is rarely useful to offer more than 10 page entries for any given item and even that is probably too many. If you have 50 entries, the reader is likely to spend more time with your index than reading the book. Also, if an entry *needs* 50 page references, it is likely that the reader will chance upon the item in question as she looks through the book.

Next, will you cite references to authors? If so, will you have a separate 'authors index' and 'subject index'? The decision will depend, to a considerable degree, on the number of other writers that you refer to. If your book is full of references to other writers, then an author index might be useful. On the other hand, if you refer to only a few other writers, you could include these in a single index, along with 'subjects'.

Publishers often indicate how long an index should be. They have to work out, when budgeting for printing, how many pages will be taken up by the index. You should note this limitation and work within it. Also, as a rule of thumb, it is a good idea to have about three index entries for every page of text. This will give you an 'average' index and, usually, a useful one.

If you decide not to make your own index, the publisher will usually arrange for this to be done for you (some publishers don't give you the option: they employ a professional straight away). If you *are* given the option to make your own index and turn it down, then you will be charged for the cost of a professional indexer's time. This can turn out to be expensive. While you are unlikely to be invoiced directly, the cost will be taken off your first royalties payment. On, then, to producing the index.

Stage one

Buy yourself a couple of 'highlighter' pens of the same colour. I suggest two in case one runs out half way through your indexing. Then, sit down with the proof copy that you have set aside for indexing. Read through it very slowly and mark up each word that you want to appear in the index. This will also mean marking up 'repeats' of words. Thus, once you have decided to index the phrase 'primary care' you must then mark up every instance of it, as it appears. This sounds difficult, but as you concentrate on it, it becomes less so. You end up with a proof copy that has between three and five 'highlighter marks' on each page. Mark, also, every subheading and every chapter heading.

Stage two

Sitting at the computer keyboard, starting at page one of the manuscript, type in each of the highlighted words and the page number on which it appears. At this stage, don't worry about the fact that they are not in alphabetical order. The beginning of your list is likely to look like this:

Health-care professionals 2

Nursing staff 2

Doctors 2

Nursing staff 3

Measles 3

Doctors 3

Stage three

Work through the entries and work on 'alternatives'. For example, the term 'health-care professionals' may also be listed as 'professionals, health care'. Make sure that you work out all the alternatives that people may look for when they are looking up a particular term. This will leave you with an extended list of words and phrases.

Stage four

Use the 'sort' feature of your word processor to put all your entries in alphabetical order. Now you will have a completed index. Check through it, a line at a time, to make sure that everything is as it should be. Sort features in word processors sometimes do some odd things and sometimes separate numbers from words. If this happens, you may have to put your index in alphabetical order by hand.

Stage five

Proof-read your index. Check that the numbers really do match up with page numbers. Spell check the index and then double-space it. Insert page numbers at the bottom of the index pages and your index is complete. Print out three copies and send two back with the proofs of the book. Keep one copy for yourself.

Index cards

The method described above is one way of making an index. Another, more traditional way, is to use sets of (appropriately named) index cards. Here, you use a separate card for each word or phrase that you decide to use in your index. You work through the book jotting down the words and phrases on the cards and noting the page numbers as you go. You then sort the cards into alphabetical order and check each card with the proofs to check that you have identified every occurrence of the word or phrase in the proofs. Finally, you type up your index from the cards, double-space the manuscript and number the pages of the index.

Proofs

Proofs are for checking and not for changing. It cannot be stressed too strongly that you cannot make changes at this stage. If you do, you are likely to be charged for the cost of resetting the pages. Check proofs, don't change them. The publisher will send you a set of symbols to use for marking up the page proofs. Learn to use them and use them clearly. If you cannot use them, make corrections clearly both in the text itself and in the margin. Although two or three other people will also read proofs, make sure that you read them thoroughly. It does neither you nor the publishers any good if the final book is full or errors (or 'typos' as they are called). Try to read the proofs carefully but quickly. I try to return proofs the day after I receive them: if this means sitting up late, then I think it is worth it.

Finally, after another long wait and after possible consultation about the cover, you will receive a pre-publication copy of your book, followed by your free copies. This is usually the best day of all. Show it to everyone, put it on the bookshelf, take it off again and admire it and then get to work on your next proposal. Meanwhile, do what you can to encourage people to buy your book. Even better, try to get people to include it on book lists for courses. Once a book is on a book list, it usually stays there. That means that for the next two or three years, students will be buying your book. That means that you make royalties.

Waiting for the reviews

Once you have got over the shock of seeing your book in print, the next wait is for reviews. Reviews usually appear between 4 and 12 months after publication. Sometimes, they don't appear at all. Magazines and journals receive huge numbers of books for review and cannot even print all the reviews that they get back from reviewers.

As ever, too, the silence of the publishers on matters relating to the book is deafening. In 1924, W.B. Maxwell wrote the following about that silence. He could have been writing this year.

> The silence of publishers is awful. An author, whether young or old, wants to know what happens when his new book appears, but rarely if ever does the publisher tell him. On the day of publication, not a word is said; on that day, week, that day fortnight, the same ominous silence is preserved.

> Another mute week passes, and the author still doesn't know if one copy or a million copies have been sold – he knows nothing until, if he is lucky, he sees an advertisement of his work saying, 'Three editions exhausted in the same number of weeks. Fourth edition binding, fifth edition printing, six edition ordered'. But even then the publisher is still silent.
>
> Maxwell 1924

You hope, obviously, for a good review and they are always the best sort. Often, though, they give you a completely different insight into your own work and a well-written review can teach you something about writing. The writer Primo Levi sums up the 'different insight' position in one of his books:

> It is known that no author deeply understands what he has written and all authors have had the opportunity of being astonished by the beautiful and awful things that the critics have found in their work and that they did not know they had put there.
>
> Levi 1989

You don't usually have to scour the journals for reviews of your book (although you probably will): the publisher will probably send you a photocopy of the review after it is published. If the review is good, the publisher will also incorporate part of the review into promotional material. They may even include a short quotation from a review on the back cover of subsequent printings of the book. In the end, though, it is difficult to know the degree to which good or bad reviews affect the sales of non-fiction books. Fifty years ago, Clifton Fadiman, a writer and book reviewer, wrote the following and it probably still applies today:

> *How influential are reviewers?* This is a hard one to answer. All the publishers' questionnaires, scientifically designed to discover just why a given book is bought, throw but a dim light on the subject, though they provide the desired quantity of statistics. Reader A buys a book because his friend B has mentioned it; that is apparently the strongest single definable factor. But this means nothing unless you know why B happened to mention it. You ask B. B replies, let us suppose, that he himself brought, read and recommended the book as the result of reading an advertisement. Now you have to find out what in that particular advertisement

caused the positive reaction to the book. Was it the
publisher's statement of the book's merits? Was it a
quotation from a reviewer? If the latter, B bought the book
because the reviewer liked it – and therefore B indirectly did
the same. The whole matter is very complex.

Fadiman 1944

Probably *any* review is better than no review at all – based on the old
show-business saying that 'it doesn't matter what they write about
you, as long as they get your name right'. The point is that a review
does draw attention to your work.

If you do get bad reviews and things begin to get you down, take
to heart, the advice offered by the writer Doris Lessing (1984):

> . . . it does no harm to repeat, as often as you can, 'Without
> me the literary agency would not exist: the publishers, the
> agents, the sub-agents, the sub-sub agents, the accountants,
> the libel lawyers, the departments of literature, the
> professors, the theses, the books of criticism, the reviewers,
> the book pages – all this vast and proliferating edifice is
> because of this small, patronised, put-down and underpaid
> person.'

Lessing 1984

Incidentally, it is almost impossible to assess, as an author (or
perhaps even as a publisher) how many of your books will sell.
Recently, one of my books on communication sold 3000 copies in a
year. Another, on a similar subject, sold 7. Was one *that* much better
(or worse) than the other?

Second editions

Make sure that you keep copies of your book manuscript on disk. If
the book sells well, the publishers may ask you to write a second
edition. Or you can suggest writing one. Second editions usually
appear about five years after the first edition.

The writing of a second edition is often more interesting than the
writing of the first. You have the chance to really get to know the
book that you wrote, to correct it where necessary and to bring it up
to date. The aim is not to write a completely new book. The second
edition should retain the 'character' and even the layout of the first.
After all, if the book is selling well, it is likely that it has become a
course book in many colleges. If lecturers are using your book to

augment their courses, they will want to know that a new edition is not too dissimilar to the first. It is usual to introduce about 25% new material into a second edition. It is also usual to retain the original title of the book.

Remember that if you refuse to prepare a second edition and the publishers are determined that one should be written, most book contracts contain a clause which states that, should the author refuse, the publishers may ask another author to write the second edition. If the second edition is written by another author and if your book has become something of a classic, your name may be retained in the title of the book. This accounts for those rather oddly titled books such as *Bacon's Textbook of Psychiatry* by Davies and Smith.

As a general rule, if you are asked to prepare a second edition, do so. Remember that you are likely to see a revival of interest in your book when the second edition comes out and that usually means an increase in sales. Sometimes, too (and for reasons that I don't understand), second editions sell better than first editions. Perhaps the phrase 'second edition', on the cover, gives the book buying public a certain confidence that the book cannot be too bad if it has run to two editions. Also, second editions usually have new covers. If you really hated the cover of your first edition, now is the time to express an interest in the colour scheme of the new one.

Before you write the second edition, you will have to write a new proposal and show the publishers how you plan to organise the work. This proposal, like the original one, will have to be approved by a publishing committee and may be sent out for review. Do not start writing the second edition until you have a contract to do so.

If your book seems to be selling well in two editions, you may want to open a series of files on your computer into which you place new material for subsequent editions. In this way, you 'live' with your book and are constantly on the lookout for new material. Given that there is nearly always a five-year gap between editions, you are going to have plenty of time to find your new material. What is particularly useful about this 'collect as you go' approach is that it allows you to keep up to date with the literature and research in the field related to your book. Also, as the author of a successful book, you are likely to be invited to give talks or conference papers on the subjects in your book. Keeping up to date is therefore essential.

Note that you are unlikely to receive an advance on royalties for second and subsequent editions and that all the above comments apply to third, fourth and fifth editions.

Editing books

If you are uncomfortable about writing or unable to write a whole book yourself, you may want to edit a book with contributions from other authors. This is by no means an easy option. In many ways, as we shall see, being the editor of a multiauthor work is more complicated than writing the book yourself. Sometimes, too, you end up virtually writing the whole book anyway.

There are certain advantages to an edited volume:

- The work is distributed among a number of writers
- There is the chance to group together 'experts' in the field
- A number of writers benefit from having their work published
- Various writers can bring variety to a book.

Be aware, though, that there are also certain disadvantages:

- Those who promise chapters may pull out later on
- Contributors may change job or leave the country
- Writers may submit their chapters late
- There may be considerable overlap in information between the chapters, which will have to be edited out
- Contributions may vary considerably in style, quality and length
- You may have to spend a considerable time on ensuring that the final work is consistent in style and quality.

It is sometimes tempting to draw together a group of friends or colleagues to work on an edited volume. If you do this, remember that, at a later date, you will have to read and critically comment on their work. This may or may not be a painful process. It may also be the case that certain friends and colleagues write really well and others do not. In this case, the ones who do not may wonder why you have singled them out for critical attention.

The secret to working on an edited volume, if there is one, is to structure the project very tightly. First, make sure that you invite only those people who you know will finish chapters and who will submit to a deadline. Second, work with all the contributors on the book proposal. Make sure that there is as little overlap as possible and that everyone knows what everyone else is writing about. Overcome any reticence you may have about asking to see potential contributors' previous work. Many people like the idea of contributing to a book but not everyone can do it. Third, prepare a set of guidelines relating to style, layout, length and so forth. Ask all contributors to stick very rigidly to these guidelines. The more structure that you can introduce at the early stages of the project, the less editing of the manuscript you are likely to have to do later on. Fourth, make sure that all contributors can send you their work on a disk and that they will be working with a word-processing program that is compatible with your own. You are going to have to edit the whole volume. If you cannot 'import' a particular chapter file into your word-processing program, you are going to have to retype it. This final point is a particularly important one. It is essential that you know, in advance, what sort of word-processing programs your contributors are going to use.

Figure 10.4 (on page 180) illustrates a set of notes that a co-editor and I sent to contributors to a multiauthor book.

The proposal for an edited volume has to be processed by the publisher in exactly the same way as a single-author book. It will be considered by a publishing committee and will be sent out for review. At this stage, of course, individual contributors' ideas may be changed by the reviewers of the proposal. At this stage, too, potential contributors may pull out of the project, having decided that the 'modified' proposal does not fall in line with their original intentions. The egos involved in multiauthor books can be very fragile! If contributors *do* pull out of the project, it falls to you to find new ones. It is always a good idea to have a 'second team' of potential authors of chapters on whom you can call if 'first team' authors pull out.

Chapter authors of edited volumes are usually paid on a 'one-off' basis. When the book is published, each author receives a single amount in payment for his or her work. You can either negotiate this figure with the authors or stipulate what it will be. Remember that all of these one-off payments will be deducted from your royalties. You will not begin to see any royalty payments from an edited volume until all the individual authors have been paid off.

Edited volumes usually take a long time to produce. As we have seen, individual authors can be slow to send you their manuscripts. What seemed like a good idea to them six months ago may become something of a burden as time goes by. The motivation for writing a single chapter is not usually as high as it is for writing a single-author book. It is useful to keep in touch with your authors and, if possible, to meet with them as a group about half way through the timespan allotted for the writing.

Once you have all the manuscripts in and you have converted the various word-processing formats to your own word-processing program, you can begin to edit. Specifically, you must edit for the following:

- Overall style
- Tense and person

Title of the book
Authors' names (eds)
We are very pleased that you have agreed to work on this project with us and we look forward very much to your chapter.

Editorial notes
These notes have been compiled to help you write your chapter and to help in maintaining a consistent style in the book. We hope they will be useful. They are only *guidelines*: don't feel too constrained by them and do come back to us for further discussion if you would like to modify them for your chapter.

Aim of the book
The book should be a readable and practical account of what it is like to do counselling in various nursing settings. Your aim should be to write a fairly personal and very practical chapter. It should not be too academic but should be appropriately referenced to the research and the literature. Don't feel, though, that you must support every statement that you make with a reference.

Market
We hope that the book will appeal to students on professional qualifications, undergraduate and counselling courses. It should also be of value to clinical nurses, nurse educators and managers.

References
Please use the Harvard system of referencing as in the following example. Please make sure that all your references are complete at the end of your manuscript.
Counselling has been widely used in intensive care settings for helping relatives to cope with grief (Brown 2003; Smith 2003).
Brown, N. 2003 *Counselling in Intensive Care*, Macmilllan, London.

Presentation of manuscript
We would be very pleased if you were able to submit your manuscript to us on a floppy disk or via e-mail in one of the following formats:

● Microsoft Word for Windows.
Don't forget to keep a copy of everything that you send to us.

Layout
Whichever of the above formats you use, please observe the following style conventions:
1. Write short sentences and short paragraphs.
2. Try to put references at the ends of sentences rather than in the middle of them.
3. Use only ONE level of subheading, in the way that we have used them in this document.
4. Paragraphing. Do not indent below a chapter heading or immediately below a subheading. Indent all subsequent paragraphs. Do not leave a further space between paragraphs. An example of a page of text in this format is included below.
5. Your manuscript should be between 5000 and 6000 words in length. Please stay within these limits.

Personal details
Please include, on a separate sheet or in a separate file, the following:
● Your full name
● Your qualifications
● A one-paragraph bibliographic note that includes your present job.

Proposal
We enclose the original proposal for this book so that you can see what the other chapters will be about.

Other points
● Try to define the *context* of your chapter very early on. If you are writing, for example, about psychiatric nursing, briefly describe when and in what circumstances counselling might be used.

Figure 10.4 Example of notes sent to contributors to a multiauthor book

- You don't have to subscribe to any particular school of counselling but try to *define* and discuss your approach.
- If you can, offer direct, practical examples of the ideas that you are discussing.
- Do try to write the 'dialogue' section of the chapter. You can base this on your own experience or, if you have them, on taped coun-selling sections. Have someone else read them through to vouch for their 'realism'.
- Do try to avoid writing too much in the 'first person'. Use 'I' when you want to refer, directly, to a personal experience but avoid using it too often.

Deadline

You can either submit the final manuscript to us or you can send a draft on which we will offer comments if these are appropriate. Deadlines are as follows:

- If you are submitting a draft: 1st December 2001
- Deadline for submission of final manuscript: 1st February 2002.

We plan to submit the final manuscript to (publisher) in June 2002.
We hope you will enjoy working on your chapter and we look forward to working with you on this exciting project. Do contact either of us at any time if you would like to talk through any aspect of your work.

Figure 10.4 *Continued*

- Grammar and spelling
- Content
- Layout.

When the going gets tough, remember that the editor *always* has the last word. If you feel strongly that something should be changed in a particular chapter, then change it. Just as you will never be completely happy with the final product when you are working on a single-author book, so you will always find problems with contributions in a multiauthor book. As I have indicated above, you may find yourself 'rewriting' the whole book. If this happens, it suggests that you have not done sufficient groundwork and planning in the early stages of the project.

Once the manuscript has been sent to the publisher, it will, again, be reviewed by external reviewers. There may, again, be suggestions for change and these changes will have to be made by individual authors. Finally, proofs will have to be read. You will be asked to do an overall proof check and each author, individually, will usually also be asked to proof-read his or her contribution. The indexing of multiauthor books is probably best left to a professional indexer. Remember that you will not 'know' the content of a multiauthor book in the way that you would a book that you wrote yourself. Personally, I would never take on the task of indexing an edited book and I have edited a few.

At the risk of sounding grim, don't take on the editing of a multiauthor book lightly. Do not see it as an easy option for getting

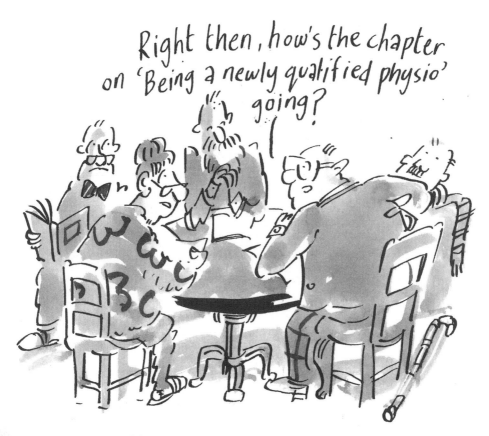

Edited works always take longer than you anticipate to compile.

into print and don't be 'talked into it' by a group of potential authors or a publisher. Only take on such a project if you really know the field well and if you have already had some editorial experience. Each time I have taken on the editing of a multiauthor text I have sworn that it would be the last time!

Writing reviews

As you write, others will ask you to review what other people have written. There are at least four reviewing possibilities:

- Book reviews
- Reviews of journal papers
- Reviews of book proposals
- Reviews of completed manuscripts.

Book reviews

Many people who work in academic departments are likely to be asked to review books for journals. If you have also published quite widely yourself, you are also likely to be asked.

The first point about book reviewing should be obvious but is not always. If you are sent a book to review, read it. It is possible to write a review by reading the 'blurb' on the back cover and flicking through the chapters. This is, however, unfair to the writer, the publisher and the readers of the journal in which the book you review is to appear. The publisher and author will immediately recognise the 'blurb review'. After all, who writes the blurb? The editor or the author.

A well-crafted review is quite difficult to write. Most people can summarise the chapters and say whether or not they liked the book. The point, though, is to offer a little more than this. The reader may also like reading book reviews. Have a look at the Sunday papers: the broadsheets contain separate review supplements and they are not there simply to sell books. They are also there because people enjoy reading them. So your review might entertain as well as guide the potential reader.

Start, perhaps, by summarising the book. Say in a few sentences what the book is about and whom it is aimed at. Then do a brief summary of the main points of the book. Close by offering an opinion on the value of the book in terms of its content, its readability and its general usefulness (or otherwise) to the potential reader.

Don't be afraid to write a 'bad' review but please remember that the author will read the review, too. As you write the review, imagine that this is your book. You have spend months working on it and are proud to see it in the shops. By all means point out the bad points of the book but I see little value in really 'panning' a book. It might be better to return it to the book review editor and suggest that you don't feel that it is an appropriate book to review. This, I accept, is a contentious view. Others take the view that the reviewer should be as 'honest' as possible and as readily damn the book as praise it. My feeling is that such an approach adds little to a book review and does not help the reader very much – except that it might give some ghoulish pleasure in seeing someone else's work torn to shreds.

Work strictly to word limits when reviewing books. You may be asked to write a review of anywhere between 100 and 5000 words. Either way, it is important to keep within those limits. If you do not, the journal will either edit your review drastically or will simply not print it.

Payment for reviewing varies from nothing at all to a few pounds. No one ever made a fortune from reviewing books (unless, of course, you become a featured book reviewer in those Sunday papers). All journals that I have come across let you keep the book that you review.

Only review books that you feel capable of reviewing. Much as you may feel flattered by being asked to review a book and might like the idea of keeping this hefty textbook that lands on your desk, only do it if it falls within your own field of expertise. To do otherwise is likely to lead to an inaccurate and not very helpful review.

Not everyone, of course, thinks that book reviewing is such a great occupation. In an interview with Robert Butler, the author and humorist Stephen Fry had this to say about reviewing:

> 'But you wouldn't want to be the one doing it, would you?'
> He offers his St Peter scenario. 'Imagine getting to the gates of heaven and St Peter says "What did you do with your life?"
>
> "Well, I spent my life looking at things that other people did and saying 'oh, I think we've seen that all before, haven't we?' And 'that's not very good'. And 'oh dear, oh dear, oh dear'."'
>
> Butler 1995

Reviews of journal papers

You may be also be invited to review other people's manuscripts sent to journals. Many health-care journals use a 'blind' peer-review process. That is to say that the writer's name is taken off the front of the manuscript before it is sent out to two reviewers who are deemed experts in the field. The journal will usually only publish papers that are accepted by both reviewers. Note, though, that the editor always has the final say in what does and what does not get published in a journal. It is possible for two reviewers to agree that a paper is worthy of publication and for the editor to decide not to accept it. Obviously, the editor has a clearer view of what is already waiting for publication and what is in keeping with the journal's policy.

If you are sent a paper for review, you will usually be sent a form to complete that has two sections: comments to the editor and comments to the writer. You will also be asked to express a view on whether or not the editor should accept the paper for publication. In recent years, some journals have begun to send out quite detailed questionnaires to their reviewers.

As you read the paper, consider, at least, the following points:

- Is the paper similar in style to other papers published in the journal?
- Is it original and does it have 'something to say'?
- If it is a research paper, have all the stages of the research process been described properly and appropriately?
- Is the layout of the paper and the reference list appropriate and complete?
- Would you recommend publication?

Be honest and constructive in your comments to the writer. This is not a time to 'score points' or to demonstrate your own knowledge of the topic in hand. It is the chance to offer valuable feedback to another person who, like you, is struggling with the writing process. If you feel that the topic discussed in the paper is beyond your expertise, don't hesitate to send the paper back with a covering letter explaining why you feel you cannot review it.

Deal with reviews of manuscripts promptly. Editors depend on a quick turnaround of papers and writers, obviously, want to be put out of their misery as quickly as possible. Do, however, make sure that you give each manuscript enough time and read it thoroughly. If necessary, write comments directly on to the manuscript as well as on the review form. Some journals pay you for your review while others do not. Normally, the 'heavyweight' journals do not pay for reviews. Either way, you learn a great deal about writing from reading other people's work and learn a considerable amount about the right and wrong ways of preparing journal papers.

Reviews of book proposals

If you have particular expertise in a particular field, you may be asked by a publisher to review a book proposal. The publisher is likely to ring or write to you first, then send you the proposal. She will ask for a report that covers the following sorts of question:

- Is there are reasonable market for a book on this topic?
- Will this sort of book have appeal in other countries? If so, which?
- Who would be the main buyers of a book like this?
- Is the author an authority in this field?
- In the case of edited books, are the contributors authorities?
- Is the contents list complete and arranged logically?
- Are there any alterations you would like to recommend?

- Which books are likely to be the main competitors with this one?
- How do you feel this book would compare with those competitors?
- Do you recommend that we should publish this book?
- Do you have any further comments?

Be fair, honest and constructive. On the one hand, the publisher will not want to publish a book that is clearly not going to sell. On the other, the potential author will appreciate constructive comments about how to improve a proposal. If you really feel that the book should not be published, outline very clearly your objections to it and the grounds for those objections. Sometimes, the publishers will send you one or more sample chapters to read and this can be a very useful indicator of the author's style. It is one thing to write a proposal and another to write the book. You are likely to receive a fee for reading and reporting on a proposal.

Reviews of completed manuscripts

If the publisher accepts your and other reviewers' comments and offers the author a contract, the book will then be written. The publishers may then approach you again to review the whole manuscript. This may also happen regardless of whether or not you reviewed the original proposal.

In these cases, you need to give the manuscript a careful, line-by-line reading for style, content, consistency, readability and accuracy. The publisher is likely to ask you for a report along the following lines:

- Is there a real need for this book and what are the likely markets for it? Please indicate the level at which the book is likely to appeal and identify the likely buyers:
  - In the United Kingdom
  - In the USA
  - Elsewhere.
- If the book has been written for the student market, how would you anticipate its being used – as a main text, as recommended reading or as 'library only'? If you can, please list likely courses.
- What would you imagine to be a reasonable price for this book?
- What are the likely competitors for this book and how do they compare with it? What particular advantages and disadvantages has the new book?

- How quickly is it likely to become out of date?
- Is the author a recognised authority in this field?
- Is the author's coverage of the material adequate and appropriate? If not, what modifications do you feel are needed?

Read the manuscript carefully and give considerable thought to your report. This is rarely the time to suggest that the manuscript needs to be rewritten from the ground up. By now, the author's proposal will have been accepted, she will have met the editor and probably kept in touch with her throughout the writing process. The end product should be very much in line with the researched proposal. If, however, you feel that it is not, don't be afraid to say so. Again, be as constructive as possible: don't 'look' for faults but do comment on them if you find them. You will receive a fee for this work and may or may not receive a copy of the book when it is published.

You can learn a very considerable amount from reading other people's proposals and manuscripts. They can teach you about other people's perceptions of the field and about how other people construct books. What you clearly cannot do, however, is to 'borrow' ideas from them. Remember that, whatever another person writes, it is copyright from the moment it is written. It does not have to be formally 'published' to make it copyright.

Finally

This chapter has identified the bones of book and review writing. I hope that it has demonstrated that writing a book is possible if you structure the process. I think it is one of the more enjoyable activities in life; I hope you will too.

To finish, I want to make a plea for sanity. The most important issue in non-fiction writing is the content. Many people find that they are so worried about style that they do not get as far as addressing the content. Sometimes, the style gets in the way and makes unclear what the content is. Start, then, with your content. Work out what it is you want to say and then write it down. I have used this method a lot with students who are worried about how to write a particular passage. I ask them to tell me what they want to write. When they have spoken, I suggest that they write down what they have said. This is nearly always the best way to write. If you can say it, you can write it.

Your aim is not to be the Joseph Conrad of essay, book and project writing. It is to convey your ideas to other people. If you stick to the basic rules of writing suggested in this book and keep your sentences and paragraphs short, you will already be some way towards effective writing.

References

Baker, J. (1987) *Copy Prep*. Blueprint, London.

Butler, R. (1995) Forever English. *The Independent on Sunday*, 12 February.

Fadiman, C. (1944) *Reading I've Liked*. Hamish Hamilton, London.

Lessing, D. (1984) Into the labyrinth. In: R. Findlater (ed.) *Author! Author!* Faber & Faber, London.

Levi, P. (1989) *Other People's Trades*. Abacus, London.

Maxwell, W.B. (1924) The sin of silence. In: R. Findlater (ed.) *Author! Author!* Faber & Faber, London.

Nelson Thornes (2003) *Author Guide*. Nelson Thornes, Cheltenham.

Reason, P. & Rowan, J. (eds) (1981) *Human Inquiry: a sourcebook of new paradigm research*. John Wiley, Chichester.

Turner, B. (ed) (1992) *The Writer's Handbook*. Macmillan/PEN, London.

Wells, G. (1989) *The Successful Author's Handbook*, 2nd edn. Macmillan, Basingstoke.

Writing: a personal view

Perhaps it is true that self-delusion most often takes the form of a belief that one can write; as to that I cannot say. My own experience has been that there is no field where one who is in earnest about learning to do good work can make such enormous strides in so short a time.

Dorothea Brande

So much for the theory. How does it all work in practice? In this chapter, I offer an illustration of the way that I write. Some books start with an introduction to the author. This one ends with one. I hope that the chapter helps to consolidate some of the issues that I have discussed in the text and also shows how, in the end, there are no immutable rules of writing. In the end, you have to find your own way. The rules, though, can help early on in structuring and making it possible to get decent marks in assignments, get articles and books published and hand in reasonable theses and research reports. Many people don't write at all because they don't know where to start.

I have been writing for publication for 20 years. During that time I have written various books – some of which have been translated into various languages – over 200 articles and papers for journals and various research reports, educational documents and many book and software reviews.

My first book was written longhand on a series of A4 pads and I found myself absorbed in the task. It took about 6 months to complete and then the handwritten manuscript was typed out by someone else. Ever since then, I have always written books on a computer and would not recommend to anyone writing a book in longhand – unless you have plenty of time and plenty of money for the typing up.

Writing the first book made the process of writing articles and papers seem easier and I went on to write more. I have also been fortunate in being asked to review other people's book proposals and their completed manuscripts. This is to be recommended. Seeing how other people work gives you lots of ideas about your own style.

Equipment and environment

I'm not fussy where I write. I have never found the need to be cloistered and to shut myself away to work. Much of my writing is done in the sitting room or dining room of our house. Other work I do on the move, while travelling. Computers seem to me to have made a difference to all this. Their portability and the fact that you can quickly switch them on and off means that you don't necessarily have to set aside a 'writing area'. Besides, we don't have the room. I have written over a period that exactly matches the growing up of my two children and I have got used to them – and various pets – being around while I work. An important point is that they can also draw you *away* from work. As far as computing is concerned, this is a good thing. It is far too easy to sit in front of a screen for far too long. Having said that, I find I write best at night and often sit up very late to finish particular projects.

At the time of writing, I use a laptop computer at home and a desktop at work. I have a laser printer at work and a 'three in one' ink jet printer at home that prints, photocopies and scans. Nothing gets on to paper before the final manuscript is finished. I don't find it useful to make lots of 'hard' (or paper) copies of things I have written and I don't keep hard copies of articles that I have sent off for publication. I do, however, keep a hard copy of book manuscripts. This is so that any editor's queries can be dealt with promptly and direct from the page. The editor, for example, sends a list of queries and all of them relate to particular pages of a manuscript. Checking these against a 'computer copy' can be difficult as page numbers sometimes get changed in the process. Working with a hard copy makes the work easier.

I use a very limited number of programs – having tried out and reviewed a great number. My word-processing program is Microsoft Word for Windows and I also use the free-form database program Idealist for storing bibliographical references. I find the combination of the two particularly useful. When I am working on an article or a book, I have both of them running under Windows. Then, when I need a reference, I can switch from Word into Idealist, look up the reference and then use 'copy and paste' features to transfer the reference from the database to the word-processing program. Over the years I have used various methods of storing bibliographical references but have found this to be the easiest and most accessible. Oddly enough, some of the most awkward programs to use are the *dedicated* referencing programs. I've never found them to have the flexibility of Idealist.

Idealist is also the program I use for collecting material for books. Its 'free-form' nature means that I can store quotations, ideas, passages of text and so on, all together in the same database. Later, I can pull out the various entries that I want as I work on the book. If I know that I will be doing a second or subsequent edition of a book, I start collecting material in this way when preliminary discussions have taken place with the publishers. If nothing comes of the idea for a new edition, I can always use the material in other ways.

Microsoft PowerPoint allows me to make various visual aids and graphical items. I use it for preparing overhead projection acetates for lecturing. I also use it for preparing graphs and other charts for research reports. Such charts can be readily copied into Word – although the word processing program also has its own, excellent, charting facility and sometimes I use that.

I have customised Word considerably. First, I have got rid of a lot of the buttons at the top of the screen that I don't use and replaced them with buttons that I do use. I have a button for counting words, another for double-spacing manuscripts, others that bring up standard templates and so on. All these things can be done from menus but I find the buttons easier to use. Also, making buttons is something that can be done during periods of lack of inspiration, while writing. It's not difficult to convince yourself that you are doing something useful when fiddling with the features of a program.

As I write, I count words. This serves two functions. First, it convinces me that I really am making progress. I used to keep a running tally of the words I had written on given days and in this way formed a view of how well (or otherwise) I was doing. Latterly, though, I find I am better at judging how much or how little I have written and better at pacing myself. I used to be a person who had to get things done as quickly as possible – a 'type A' personality, if you like. Illness and a tendency to burnout have meant that I have slowed down and learned to be a bit more moderate in my writing habits. The second reason for counting words is to make sure that I am within the word allocation afforded by publishers or journal editors. It's no use sending in a journal paper of 6000 words when the limit is 2500. One of the real high spots in writing is edging up towards the final word limit of a book manuscript. Sometimes, the anticipation of it causes a sudden drop off of inspiration. It's a bit like being an athlete and seeing the tape in front of you and suddenly feeling your legs buckling. If I sense this happening, I use rather elaborate ploys to pretend that I am not 'really' nearing the target. I stop counting words or I treat the final section as though it were an essay on its own. Or I practise 'thought blocking' if I find myself thinking about the last few thousand words. Generally the first and last 2000 words of any book are the most difficult ones to write.

The writing routine

First, it *is* a routine. I try to write something every day and aim at finishing something for publication at least every month. In between times, there are various other writing projects, some work-related and others to do with reviews of books and manuscripts. I am quite sure that I would not want to be a full-time writer. It is the 'other' work that I do that feeds the writing and I can't imagine what it must be like to get up and come downstairs to a cold computer every morning. Teaching and travelling I find particularly rewarding in relation to writing. Both spark off new ideas and encourage the seeing of things from different perspectives.

When writing articles, I usually write the whole thing in my head, before sitting down at the keyboard. I rarely write 'commissioned' pieces and find these difficult. Instead, most of the articles that I write stem from ideas that I have thought about while working. Very often, the 'whole' of the plan for an article – and sometimes for a book – arrives in one 'lump'. Then, it is a question of teasing out the various points, working out headings and subheadings and deciding at whom the piece should be aimed. I have found it useful to learn about the various house styles of different publications and then work on an article with that publication in mind. I also try to imagine the readership of a given piece although this is such an abstract idea that I am not sure that it really works.

Once I have the piece written in my head, I transfer it to the computer. I write quickly, at first, and don't stop to correct mistakes. The first draft is always a sort of 'stream of consciousness' piece, although as time has gone on I have found it easier to structure the writing as it goes into the computer. Sometimes, I write down a series of headings before I start but, more often, I return to put the headings in later. Even in the first draft I make sure that there are lots of paragraph breaks and use the layout of the notebook computer to help in this respect. If I have been writing for some time and cannot see any paragraph breaks on the part of the screen that is visible, I go back and insert some. It seems to me that short sentences and short paragraphs really are the basis of effective writing.

Once I have written the first draft of an article, I spell-check it. I never used to be any good at spelling but, ironically, the spell-checker has made me a better one. By being presented, on a regular basis, with the same old errors of spelling, I have begun to absorb the correct spellings. Now, I try to beat the spell-checker.

The spell-checker takes care of some of the grosser problems with the original draft. Next, I work through the paper, a paragraph at a time, and rework each one. This is the stage, too, in which I put in references. During the writing of the first draft, I merely leave three asterisks in brackets – i.e. (***) – to indicate where references should go. I always try to make sure that references go at the ends of sentences so that the reader is not distracted by a sudden outpouring of odd names and dates. The insertion of references often leads to new ideas for certain paragraphs or sections. Recalling what other writers or researchers have said leads, often, to further debate about particular issues.

I try to make the second draft the final one. The idea that your work necessarily improves the more you work on it doesn't seem to match my experience. I have found it possible to 'polish to death' a piece of writing and thus remove any sort of spontaneity or life from it. After all, the process is not a scientific one and I don't believe that you can continue to hone down a piece of writing until it approaches the ideal. All writing is something of a compromise and, looking back, I realise that some pieces I have written have been more of a compromise than others. In the end, though, it doesn't pay to be too hard on yourself. Most of us are not in the business of producing works of art. The main thing, presumably, is to communicate ideas to others in as clear a way as possible. To this end, and in the second draft, I further check sentence and paragraph length and insert headings if they are not already there. I also try to take out big words and lighten the more leaden passages. I also trim out as many of the 'however's and 'there is a sense in which's as I can find. Most writing benefits from trimming in this way.

Sometimes, I run the grammar-checking feature of the word processor. This checks for, at least, the following: spelling, tense, over-long sentences, basic errors of grammar. It also offers a summary of the 'readability' of the text. I don't use this as a matter of course but when I am working on something very different or new or when I am writing for a particular journal that requires a particular style. Sometimes, too, the thesaurus feature of the word processor can be useful in finding alternative words.

The last thing I do with articles is to make sure that they are double-line spaced (although I work in single-line spacing 'on the screen'), page-numbered and have a title page. I also pay a lot of attention to the general layout of the words on the page. I never use 'justified right' margins but leave them 'ragged' as this makes manuscripts easier to read. I also make sure that the spacing between headings and text is uniform and check, again, for typos. Obviously, spell-checkers can miss some less obvious errors such as the inappropriate uses of 'two', 'to' and 'too'.

I used to ask my wife to read articles before I sent them off but do not do so now. About five years ago she got fed up with reading them. Instead, I sometimes ask work colleagues to read them through and then make some changes. If I do this, I make them copies and ask them to write their comments directly on to the appropriate pages. This makes it easier to sit at the computer keyboard and make changes directly to the text.

Like everyone else, the articles that I send off are either accepted, rejected out of hand or sent back for modification. I try to deal with the latter as soon as possible and always send a covering letter enumerating the changes that have been made. This is done in the probably erroneous belief that the editor will be pleased that I have made exactly the changes that were asked for. My experience with editors is that it mostly pays to do what you are told. Either that, or the editor can reject your work. In arguing, you may have scored on some sort of point of principle but you don't get to see your paper in print. This is not to suggest that I am some sort of doormat but I hope to acknowledge that nothing that anyone writes is so important that it cannot be changed.

Writing books

Books take much more structuring than do articles. You can't just sit down at a blank screen and start typing page 1 – at least, not for a non-fiction book. When planning a book, again, I usually find that the idea for the book 'arrives' as a whole. Then, in my head, I separate out the various chapters. For a book of about 50,000 words, I usually aim at 10 chapters and this becomes 12 or 14 for a book of up to 100,000 words.

I work out a fairly detailed book proposal, including a rationale for the book, a review of some competing books, details of the various chapters and information about when the manuscript will be delivered and how long it will be. I then send it to an editor at a publisher and often I will have discussed it with that editor before I send it off. As is the case with articles, the response is the same: outright rejection, outright acceptance or acceptance subject to major or minor changes.

This time, though, there are a couple of stings in the tail. First, the proposal is sent out, by the editor, to various reviewers and this process can take a long time. By the time the reviews come in, it is sometimes possible to have rethought your position about a particular book that you have planned. Fortunately, new ideas can usually be incorporated into the manuscript. Second, the reviewers review anonymously. That gives some reviewers licence to say exactly what they think about a proposal and some don't mince words at all. You can usually tell, from the editor's covering letter that comes to you with the reviewer's comments, that there are some 'bad' ones. In these cases, the editor will often write something like 'Don't be too put off by some of the comments: I feel that they are meant constructively'. I always am put off by them, though. It has taught me, if nothing else, to be careful what I write when reviewing other people's proposals. Either way, if there are lots of negative responses to a proposal, the editor will, rightly, have to decide whether or not to accept a proposal or to ask for very radical changes.

It isn't an exact science, though. I had one proposal turned down outright by one publisher. I then sent a very slightly modified version of it to another publisher, a year later. The second publisher offered me a contract and the book went on to sell more than any of my other books.

One thing is essential: that all royalty statements and payment advice slips from publishers are kept for tax purposes. A good year, in royalties terms, means a bad year the following year when the tax has to be paid. Tax returns are prepared every April and the tax bill is paid in the January and July of the following year.

Some manuscripts have to be submitted as 'camera-ready copy': what you see on the page is what I have typed on my computer. This process is painfully intense but gets easier the more you do it. The publishers that ask for copy to be prepared in this way lay down very particular standards for margin settings, page numbering, indexing and so on.

Writing the book

Once a contract has been received and signed, I prepare the complete outline of the book in the following way. The process has become a sort of ritual. First, I open up a new directory on a computer. The directory, for this book, is called 'Write'. Then, I open up a series of new files, within that directory, to correspond to each of the chapters and sections of the book. Thus, apart from files for the chapters, there will be files for references, a bibliography and any appendices that are planned. In each of these files, I prepare the chapter heading and – as far as possible – all the main sub-headings.

I also set up any 'macros' or computerised short-cuts that will be useful during the writing of the book. Macros can be a useful way of making sure that all parts of the book are uniform.

The structuring of an outline in this way and the preparation of the computer is an important part of the writing process. It gives me confidence that I really can finish the book and it gives me an idea of where everything is to go and what sections need further research.

At this time, I also prepare a series of envelope files to correspond to each of the proposed chapters. I use these to file away odd notes, photocopies of articles and anything else that will be useful. I mark these up with a thick marker pen to indicate the chapter number and the title of the chapter. In this way, I can quickly pull out the appropriate file. I would like to be able to say that these are then neatly filed away but they are not. They sit on the printer or – more usually – on the floor until the book is finished. Obviously, not everything gets used but it becomes tempting to adopt a squirrel approach during the writing of a book.

The other pile that tends to develop is a pile of books, which becomes bigger as the book progresses. Towards the end of a book, I tend to find that I have received more than my fair share of 'overdue books' notices from various libraries. These three sources of information – the envelope files containing papers, the Idealist database containing notes and the pile of books – tend to be the most frequently referred to sources during writing.

The computer files can be brought together, at any time, in Word, using the feature 'Masterfile'. This is a file that can automatically draw together all the other files so that it is possible to see what the whole book will look like. It is also useful, of course, when printing out the final manuscript. Incidentally, WordPerfect has a similar but much better masterfile feature.

Over the next few months, the book gets written. I work on it most days and 'live' with it all the time. I am reminded of a friend who was having psychoanalysis and who found himself dealing with the topic of 'anxiety' during one period of his analysis. During that period, he talked of nothing else. Similarly, when I am working on a book on a particular topic, I find myself caught up in noticing anything to do with that topic that appears in the press or on television. Fortunately, I have not yet got to the stage when it becomes the only topic of conversation too.

I tend to work for long periods once I get going. If I hit a real purple patch I can find myself sitting at the computer for four or five hours at the weekends. This is not to be recommended and I am working on cutting this down. Not only can it lead to problems with wrist joints but it's not particularly good for the circulation, either. It is particularly bad for family life.

I spell-check at the end of every session and word-count. I also make double backups of everything. First, I back-up any new work to the tape streamer. Second, I back-up the chapters to a single floppy disk. Since the major hard disk crash, this is something I never skimp on. Most people have heard of horror stories in which people lost the whole of a PhD thesis from a computer and I have no particular desire to join their ranks with a book manuscript, although I have lost whole chapters early in my computer career.

I don't necessarily write the chapters in the order in which they appear in the book. I tend to start with an 'easy' chapter in order to get started. Then I try to get the difficult ones written while I am still reasonably fresh. I like to finish on an easy one, although the last things written are usually the conclusion and the introduction. The main difficulty is always retaining a consistency in writing style and trying not to repeat yourself. It is also important that chapters are roughly the same length and have roughly the same number of subsections. I also think that it is helpful to have about the same number of references at the end of each chapter.

Once the whole draft manuscript is completed in chapter form, I bring all the chapters together in one big file. From then on, I work with the whole manuscript. This is not as difficult as it sounds as I make a lot of use of the 'bookmark' feature of Word. The program allows you to insert labelled bookmarks at any point in the manuscript. These bookmarks can then be accessed, instantly, from a menu that can be pulled up on the screen. I make a bookmark for each of the chapter headings and then add others as the need arises. Working with the whole manuscript seems to increase the likelihood of consistency in style and layout.

There comes a point when you have to stop. The tendency is to want to keep working on a manuscript, feeling that there must be numerous ways in which it could be improved. There are, of course, but just sitting looking at the thing for months on end and tinkering with it are not going to guarantee quality. At some point, you decide the book is finished. Then, there are numerous checks.

The first check is for layout. Here, all the chapter headings and subheadings are checked for font size, emphasis and spacing. This may be overkill but I am a bit obsessive about such things. The second check is for the references. I run a 'search' command on an open bracket – (– and this takes me to each reference in turn. Using the 'window split' feature of Word, in which two parts of the same document can appear on the screen at the same time, I check each reference against the reference list at the end of each chapter or at the end of the book. The third check is the reference list itself. I make sure that all the references are in the correct format and that book titles and journal titles are italicised. I also check that publishers and place of publication are complete.

Finally, the whole manuscript gets a final, on-screen read through and edit and then gets printed out. I print three copies: two for the publisher and one for keeping for checking the editor's queries. Then the two copies go off to the publisher in a large padded bag along with a disk copy or the files by e-mail.

There is a sense of let-down on completion of the manuscript. Having lived with it for a number of weeks or months, there is a bit of a gap and a long wait. The publisher, during this time, has sent the manuscript out to a referee to read and comment on it. It is unusual to be asked to do major surgery on the manuscript after this reading but it can happen. Once the referee has commented, the book goes to a copy-editor, who checks the whole manuscript for style, consistency, spelling, grammar and so on. All these stages are described in Chapter 10.

Answers to editors' queries can sometimes throw up a second list of queries. Once the copy-editor has seen your answers, she sometimes (and appropriately) asks 'If you have said *this* on page 34, can you say *that* on page 89? Please clarify.' Copy-editors' queries are always terse and always remind me of teachers' notes on the bottom of school essays. One day, a copy-editor is going to write 'See me' at the bottom of a list of queries. For all that, a lot can be learned from responding to these queries and a lot more from seeing the copy-editor's final marking up of the manuscript. Much of what was originally written has been crossed out, changed or rewritten in some way and nearly always (in my experience) for the better.

The relationship between a copy-editor and a writer is a strange one. While I have received letters from them, lists of queries and phone calls, I have yet to *meet* one. It is like having a slightly detached pen-friend: the relationship, though, is short and sometimes intense.

Another long wait and then the proofs come for correction. I try to deal with these by return, although also due at this time is the index. I have explained in the text how an index is prepared and it is a process that I quite enjoy. I don't enjoy proof-reading, though, and I suspect that I am not very good at it. On the other hand, it is not a job to be skimped. Nor is a task that anyone else is likely to take on for you, for love or money.

Finally, the book comes out. Sometimes, I will have had a glimpse of this before it happens. Some publishers negotiate on issues of cover colour and design. Others don't. Then, the first you know of what a book will look like is when you open the copy that is sent to you. On rare occasions, the book gets into the shops before you are sent a copy and then you have to have a good look at it there.

Then the longest wait of all: waiting for reviews. Sometimes, of course, there aren't any. At least that saves you from the bad ones. For some reason or other, I always seem to find reviews in journals on the shelves of newsagents. If the reviews are less than glowing, I'm depressed for the rest of the day. How actors go back on stage after a night of bad notices, I don't know. On the other hand, a good review can leave you manic for a week. The worst, possibly, are the ones that are simply a summary of the blurb on the back cover. If you write reviews, please remember that the author also reads them. I know, traditionally, that everyone is supposed to be very adult and objective about this and no one wants a bad book to get a good review, but – please – just choose your words carefully. You're treading on someone's keyboard, as it were.

This, then, is how I write. It may not suit you. It doesn't always suit me. Nor does it do to *stick* to a routine. Every so often it is important to experiment a little and to do things differently. My aim is to write a novel. A colleague once remarked that my books already contain enough fiction. Good luck with your own writing.

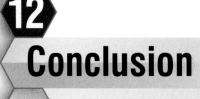

12 Conclusion

> It is a commonplace that every writer must turn to himself
> to find most of his material.
>
> Dorothea Brande

This book has been about all aspects of the writing process. In this last chapter, I have attempted to summarise the important points about any sort of writing.

- **Use STRUCTURE**. Structure the way in which your work is written (by using headings and subheadings). Also structure the way you work. Break down larger projects into sections, use time in an organised way and limit the amount of time you sit and write. Don't attempt to write large projects at one sitting.

- **Remain SIMPLE in your writing**. This has been a theme all the way through this book and it remains as a closing one. It is far better to keep your writing simple – whatever the project. Simple writing is better in both academic work and in the process of writing novels. Use short sentences and paragraphs, do not use complicated punctuation, avoid Latin and other 'foreign' words where possible and make sure that any reader will understand what you have written.

- **Keep a REFERENCE system**. You must have a database that contains references to other authors' work. This can be a card file or a computerised system. Whatever system you use, keep it up to date. Do not rely on your memory alone. Make backups of your reference files if you use a computerised system.

- **Use a COMPUTER with which to write**. Once you have learned to use a word-processing package, write directly to the computer. Do not write your work out longhand and then transfer it to the computer. Instead, write quickly to the computer and edit slowly once you have written the bulk of your project.

- **Use the SPELL-CHECKER** and, if in doubt, the grammar-checker in your word-processing package. Both, ironically, will help to improve your spelling and grammar.

- **COUNT WORDS**: whatever the project, make sure that you know how many words you have written. Checking them as you write will act as a reinforcer: every time you write a bit more, you will be nearer your target. Most writing projects involve writing to a certain limit. If you are writing for publication or a dissertation or thesis, it is vital that you do not exceed these limits.

- **Make sure that you READ**. As was noted at the beginning of this book, other people's words are the fuel for your own. Read widely, read novels and do not simply stick to the work that has been published in your own discipline. If you are a nurse, read medical journals. If you are an occupational therapist, read nursing journals, and so on. Read posters, packets and newspapers. Read for style as well as for content. In particular, get to know about various journals' and publishing companies' house styles.

- **Pay attention to LAYOUT**. A well-laid-out essay, manuscript or thesis can make a considerable 'psychological' difference to the reader. This is not to say that good layout can cover up bad work but to note that a well-produced piece of work is generally easier and more pleasurable to read. Keep the layout simple and structured and use one (or, at the most, two) types of font or typeface. If you are preparing essays, manuscripts, dissertations or theses, make sure that you double-line-space your work.

- **Use DIAGRAMS and FIGURES sparingly**. Make each one earn its keep. In particular, do not be tempted to present the findings of quantitative research as a series of tables, unlinked by prose. Most people get 'number blind' very quickly. Choose the right sort of diagram or figure to represent what it is you are trying to convey. Remember, too, that diagrams and figures should be used in place of prose: they should, as far as possible 'speak for themselves'.

- **PRACTISE writing**. If you can, write every day. If not, write regularly and notice the development of your own style. Ask other people for feedback on your work. If you write for publication you will get this anyway. Be prepared to feel quite sensitive about reading other people's comments about your work but note what they have to say and then get back to writing.

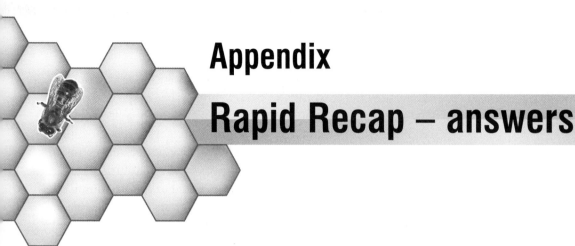

Appendix

Rapid Recap – answers

Chapter 1

1. List three things which help the presentation of your writing.

1. Paper quality, page layout, typeface used, line spacing, number of paragraphs per page.

2. List four ways to improve your writing style.

2. Use short sentences where possible, vary the sentence length, avoid complicated punctuation, avoid jargon where possible, avoid empty phrases to pad your work out, write as you would speak.

3. When might you see the use of 'sic'?

3. In a direct quote to denote that there is a grammatical or spelling error by the original author.

Chapter 2

1. What are the most important pieces of basic equipment when doing a significant amount of writing?

1. Computer, desk, comfortable chair, sticky notes to write on.

Chapter 3

1. What are the four main types of computer?

1. Desktop, laptop, notebook, palmtop.

2. What does RAM stand for?

2. Random access memory.

3. Why is it important to install a firewall on your computer?

3. To prevent viruses from attaching to your machine (often from the Internet) and corrupting or deleting programs.

Chapter 4

1. What is a macro?

1. A shorthand program that allows a function to be performed by a simple one or two keystrokes, e.g. backing up to floppy disk by pressing ALT D.

2. What is a sans serif font?

2. A font in which the letters don't have 'tails'.

Chapter 5

1. List three reasons a writer should keep a database.

1. Storing and retrieving interview data; storing and retrieving numerical data; keeping odd bits of information that are not easily classified; storing ideas for papers, articles, research projects and books; storing quotable quotes; analysing qualitative data; storing and retrieving names and addresses; keeping track of a project; collecting and executing 'to do' lists.

2. What are the six fields recommended for a simple reference database?

2. Surname and initials of author, year of publication, title, publisher and place of publication, keywords, comments.

Chapter 6

1. What does OHT stand for?

1. Overhead transparency.

2. List three ways of preparing your notes for giving a presentation.

2. Index cards (numbered), colour code cards along with visual aids, staple sheets together but take non-stapled too, format your speech into bite-sized chunks of text, which allows you to present it and breathe in the right places too!

Chapter 7

1. What does 'brainstorming' mean?

1. Jotting down, in any order as they come to you, all the words and associations related to a question or issue.

2. List three ways of collecting information for an essay.

2. Borrowing library books; using your own books and those referred to within them; looking through library bibliographical volumes; looking through CD-ROMs of bibliographies.

3. What is meant by the term 'plagiarism'?

3. The attempt to pass off someone else's written work as your own, i.e. copying straight out of books, articles and papers into your own work.

Chapter 8

1. What is the difference between a dissertation and a thesis?

1. A dissertation is what undergraduates write in their final year and what masters students write as part of the requirements for their degree. A thesis is what doctoral students hand in as the final report of their research. Note: in the USA and Canada the labels are reversed.

2. What is the difference between a reference list and a bibliography?

2. A reference list is a listing of all of the works you have directly referred to in your dissertation or thesis. A bibliography is a separate listing of other books that are related to the topic but are not referred to in your work.

3. What support can you expect from your dissertation/thesis supervisor?

3. Clear guidance on how to proceed with a particular part of your study; regular feedback on any written work that you hand in; help with methodology and analysis; guidance on how to write up your project; support and interest; regular meetings.

4. What can your supervisor expect from you?

4. Regular written reports; motivation; ability to work independently; awareness of how to use the method that you have chosen; realistic aims that you negotiate together.

Chapter 9

1. Name two different types of article in your professional magazine.

1. Short research report; example of good practice; historical article; short, controversial piece; case study; discussion of current theory; practice debate.

2. What happens in a blind refereeing system?

2. Your work is sent to two peers in your field without their knowing your name.

Chapter 10

1. What are the main stages in writing a book?

1. Completing the outline, doing the research, doing the writing, preparing the manuscript, sending it to the publishers, waiting, dealing with queries, the author's questionnaire and proof-reading, and preparing the index.

2. As a co-editor of a book, what should you look for in terms of editing contributors' material?

2. Overall style (is it consistent with the rest of the book?), tense and person, grammar and spelling, content and layout.

3. As a journal reviewer, what questions should you ask yourself when reading a paper?

3. Is the paper similar in style to other papers published in the journal? Is it original and does it have 'something to say'? If it is a research paper, have all the stages of the research process been described properly and appropriately? Is the layout of the paper and the reference list appropriate and complete? Would you recommend publication?

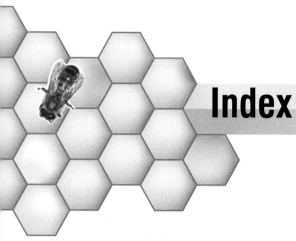

Index